ALZHEIMER'S DISEASE

LICENSE, DISCLAIMER OF LIABILITY, AND LIMITED WARRANTY

ALZHEIMER'S DISEASE

Alia Bucciarelli, MS

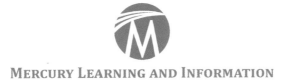

MERCURY LEARNING AND INFORMATION

Dulles, Virginia
Boston, Massachusetts
New Delhi

Publisher: David Pallai
MERCURY LEARNING AND INFORMATION
22841 Quicksilver Drive
Dulles, VA 20166
info@merclearning.com
www.merclearning.com
(800) 232-0223

This book is printed on acid-free paper.

Alia Bucciarelli. *Alzheimer's Disease.*
ISBN: 978-1-93758553-2

Library of Congress Control Number: 2015934532
161718432   Printed in the United States of America

Our titles are available for adoption, license, or bulk purchase by institutions, corporations, etc. For additional information, please contact the Customer Service Dept. at (800)232-0223(toll free).

All of our titles are available in digital format at authorcloudware.com and other digital vendors. Companion disc files for this title are available by contacting info@merclearning.com. The sole obligation of MERCURY LEARNING AND INFORMATION to the purchaser is to replace the disc, based on defective materials or faulty workmanship, but not based on the operation or functionality of the product.

To my grandfather, David Goldberg.

Contents

Alzheimer's Disease Prescription Drug Treatment

Alzheimer's Disease Nondrug Treatment

Living with Alzheimer's Disease

Being a Caregiver

Planning Ahead

Acknowledgments

Several people contributed directly or indirectly to this book. I sincerely thank Jenny Figueroa and Lavonne Beckford for sharing their caregiving experiences with me with candor and grace; it is their mother, Violet, upon whom the opening vignettes are based. I also thank Madeline Siedler, who provided me research and writing support, for which I am grateful. Finally, I thank my husband and children for their love.

Credits

Chapter Opener Figure Credits

Chapter 1- "Cerebral lobes" by derivative work of this - Gutenberg Encyclopedia.
   Licensed under CC BY-SA 3.0 via Wikimedia Commons

Chapter 2- "PET-image" by Jens Maus (http://jens-maus.de/) - Own work. Licensed under Public
   Domain via Wikimedia Commons

Chapter 3- License CC0 Public Domain

Chapter 4- © by Daniel Sone (Photographer)

Chapter 5- © by Ray Nata - Own work. Licensed under GFDL via Wikimedia Commons

Chapter 6- © by Sigismund von Dobschütz - Own work. Licensed under CC BY-SA 3.0 via
   Wikimedia Commons

Chapter 7- © by I Craig from Glasgow, Scotland - Birthday Cake

Chapter 8- © by Department of Foreign Affairs and Trade - Operation Open Heart.
   Licensed under CC BY 2.0 via Wikimedia Commons

Chapter 9- © by Alex Proimos from Sydney, Australia - The Fountain of Youth.
   Licensed under CC BY 2.0 via Wikimedia Commons

Introduction

In this book, we follow Violet and her daughters on their journey with Alzheimer's disease. As of the publishing of this book, Violet, who was diagnosed seven years ago, is 82 years old. She lives in an elder care facility, where she is safe and cared for by a team of professionals. Her husband lives around the corner, in the house in which they raised their four daughters.

She and her family have learned a lot on this journey, certainly about Alzheimer's disease, but also about aging, loving, and living.

In this book, you will learn key, practical information about Alzheimer's disease, including what its symptoms are, how it is diagnosed, what treatments are available, how to manage challenging behavior, and how caregivers can take care of themselves. But you'll also get a sense of what it is like for people with Alzheimer's disease and their families as they move through the disease, from the first early symptoms to the final days.

Although Alzheimer's disease was identified more than 100 years ago, it is only within the last 30 years that research into the disease has gained momentum. Much is left to discover, including the exact biological changes that cause it and how to reverse, slow, or prevent it.

If you think you or someone you love has Alzheimer's disease, talk with your doctor or theirs. But remember that you are not alone. There are many excellent doctors who specialize in treating people with Alzheimer's disease, and there are many excellent support groups to guide and support you.

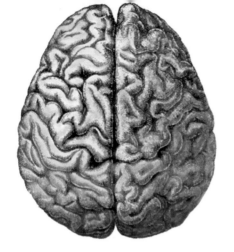

Alzheimer's Disease Basics •——

Case Study

In the evenings, after the desert heat had dissipated but before the sun had set, you could find Violet gardening in her front yard. Wife, mother of four, and grandmother of 6, Violet could coax the plum tree in the center of her yard into bloom despite the Arizona desert climate. She always had a story or joke to share with the neighbors and was the first person they would ask about the local goings-on. When she wasn't gardening, she was babysitting her grandkids, helping them with their homework, and cooking them food from her native Jamaica.

It wasn't long after she turned 73 that Violet began to become forgetful. Disorganization and trouble making decisions followed. At first, her daughters and husband thought that she was just getting quirky as she aged. But when her memory problems worsened, her daughters took her to see a doctor. They knew something was wrong, but they didn't suspect Alzheimer's disease. Looking back, Violet's daughters wish they had known what Alzheimer's disease was and how it affected the brain so that they could have recognized their mother's symptoms, sought help earlier, and begun planning for her care right away.

1. What is Alzheimer's disease?

Alzheimer's disease is a progressive disease that affects the brain. The first symptoms of Alzheimer's disease develop slowly. They are usually memory loss and confusion. But over time, symptoms worsen and begin to include changes in

DEFINITION Simply put, Alzheimer's disease is a disease that damages the brain over time, causing problems with memory, thinking, and behavior.

personality and behavior. Ultimately, people with the disease lose the ability to function on their own and need total care. There is neither a cure nor a treatment to prevent or delay the inevitable progression of the disease.

Americans fear Alzheimer's disease even more than cancer.

NOTE

Alzheimer's disease and its symptoms are not a part of normal aging. Some people may mistakenly think so, however, because Alzheimer's disease symptoms start after age 65 in most people.

For a video with Alzheimer's expert Dr. Nina Silverberg from the National Institute on Aging about what Alzheimer's disease is, visit the website of the National Institute on Aging at

ON THE WEB

http://nihseniorhealth.gov/videolist.html#alzheimersdisease.

As we age, changes take place in all parts of our bodies, including the brain. This is normal. Some people find that it takes them longer to learn new things, that they don't retain information as well as they used to, or that they lose or misplace items like their keys or glasses. Although these signs of mild forgetfulness may be annoying, they are not serious memory problems. In people with Alzheimer's disease, however, what seems like simple forgetfulness at first eventually becomes trouble thinking clearly and doing everyday tasks like shopping, driving, and cooking. Over time, people with Alzheimer's disease need someone to take care of even their most basic needs, including feeding, bathing, and dressing.

2. Where did the name "Alzheimer's disease" come from?

The disease is named after Dr. Alois Alzheimer, a German doctor (see Figure 1.1). In 1906 he described the case of a woman who

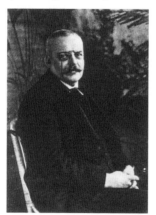

had died of an unusual mental illness that included memory loss, language problems, and unpredictable behavior. In the autopsy of her brain, he noted that she had abnormal brain tissue. In 1910 a colleague of Dr. Alzheimer's, Emil Kraepelin, called this condition "Alzheimer's disease" in his book, *Psychiatrie*, which classified and described psychiatric disorders.

◄ FIGURE 1.1
Dr. Alois Alzheimer, who first described Alzheimer's disease

A healthy brain has billions of **nerve cells (neurons)**. These cells have long branches that extend out from them. The places where the branches connect to other nerve cells are called "**synapses**."

These connections enable information to travel throughout the brain and form the basis for memories, thoughts, sensations, emotions, movements, and skills.

 For an interactive tour of how the brain works and is affected by Alzheimer's disease, visit Inside the Brain: An Interactive Tour from the Alzheimer's Association at

http://www.alz.org/alzheimers_disease_4719.asp

Broadly, Alzheimer's disease causes nerve cells and synapses in the brain to stop working and eventually die.

Experts think that Alzheimer's disease begins to damage the brain 20 or more years before symptoms become noticeable. This period of time is sometimes called the "preclinical stage" of Alzheimer's disease. Preclinical means before symptoms can be observed and diagnosed.

The three main hallmarks in the brain of Alzheimer's disease are:

- **Beta-amyloid plaques**—clumps made up of bits of protein, brain cells, and nerve cells in the space between brain cells
- **Neurofibrillary tangles**—build-up of a protein called "tau" inside nerve cells
- Loss of synapses between brain cells

Amyloid plaques and neurofibrillary tangles tend to spread in the brain in a predictable pattern. For example, they first start to form in areas of the brain involved in learning and memory and in thinking and planning. Then they spread to areas involved in speaking and understanding speech.

Brain cells can't live when they lose their connections to other brain cells. As these cells die, the brain starts to shrink (see Figure 1.2).

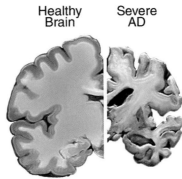

Healthy Brain   Severe AD

➤ **FIGURE 1.2**
Effect on the brain of severe Alzheimer's disease.

SOURCE: Image courtesy of the National Institute on Aging/National Institutes of Health

As damage spreads throughout the brain, symptoms worsen (see Figure 1.3).

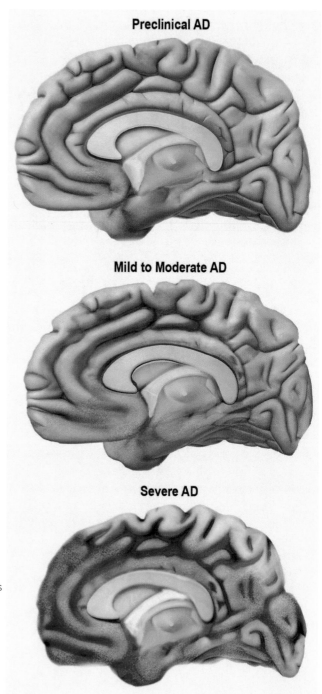

Preclinical AD

Mild to Moderate AD

Severe AD

➤ **FIGURE 1.3**
Spread of Alzheimer's disease in the brain.

SOURCE: Image courtesy of the National Institute on Aging/National Institutes of Health

4. What is early-onset Alzheimer's disease?

In rare cases, people develop Alzheimer's disease in their 30s, 40s, or 50s. When this occurs, it is called "early-onset" Alzheimer's disease. In some cases, early-onset Alzheimer's disease is caused by an abnormal change ("mutation") in one of three different inherited genes. This is called "familial" Alzheimer's disease.

ON THE WEB

For a video that shows how Alzheimer's affects the brain, watch "Inside the Brain: Unraveling the Mystery of Alzheimer's Disease" from the Alzheimer's Disease Education and Referral Center of the National Institute on Aging at

http://www.nia.nih.gov/alzheimers/alzheimers-disease-video.

Despite the younger age at which it strikes, early-onset Alzheimer's disease progresses and affects the brain in the same way as the more common late-onset Alzheimer's disease.

5. What is late-onset Alzheimer's disease?

Nine out of ten people with Alzheimer's disease develop symptoms when they are age 65 or older. When this occurs, it is called "late-onset" Alzheimer's disease. Unlike the case with early-onset Alzheimer's disease, the exact cause of late-onset Alzheimer's disease is still unclear. But experts think that genes, environment, and lifestyle may play roles.

6. How common is Alzheimer's disease?

Estimates vary of how many people in the United States have Alzheimer's disease. But experts think it is about five million people, or one in nine people age 65 and older and one in three people age 85 and older. But because it is underdiagnosed, only half of those who have the disease may know it.

In 2015, about 473,000 people will develop Alzheimer's disease in the United States; about half will be age 85 and older.

More women than men have Alzheimer's disease. Nearly two-thirds of people with Alzheimer's disease are women. This is because women live longer than men and older age increases the risk of the disease. However, men and women are equally likely to develop Alzheimer's disease at the same age.

NOTE

Because of increases in the proportion of Americans age 65 and older, the number of people who develop Alzheimer's disease each year will double by 2050.

Alzheimer's disease is the sixth leading cause of death in the United States, with about 83,000 deaths a year, according to death certificates. But Alzheimer's disease and other forms of dementia are often not reported on death certificates, and some experts think that the number of people who die from Alzheimer's disease is actually much higher, maybe even five times higher.

Dementia is an overall term for disorders that cause changes in how people behave, think, and process information.

7. How is Alzheimer's disease related to mild cognitive impairment?

Mild cognitive impairment (MCI) is a condition in which people have more memory problems than normal for their age but are still able to manage their daily activities. Cognitive means having to do with activities such as thinking, understanding, learning and remembering.

Up to one out of every five people age 65 or older has mild cognitive impairment (MCI), but not everyone with the condition will go on to develop dementia.

Symptoms of MCI are noticeable to the person who has them and to their loved ones. They include:

- Misplacing items a lot
- Missing important events or appointments
- Forgetting words

People with MCI are more likely than those without it to later develop Alzheimer's disease. Among those who see a doctor about symptoms of MCI, nearly half go on to develop some form of dementia in three or four years. But in some people, MCI remains stable or resolves on its own.

Many experts think that when someone goes on to develop dementia, the MCI was an early stage of that dementia, rather than a separate condition. Studies are in progress to learn more about why some people with MCI do and others don't develop dementia.

Cognitive function is the ability to think, remember, and reason.

People who have symptoms of MCI should see a doctor right away to find out what the cause is and possibly to treat it.

8. How is Alzheimer's disease related to dementia?

About 14 percent of people age 71 years and older in the United States have some form of dementia.

Dementia is caused by damage to the nerve cells in the brain. A number of diseases or conditions can trigger this damage, and the rate at which symptoms progress varies. In fact, different types of dementia tend to have different patterns of symptoms and changes in the brain.

Many people, especially those who are 80 years and older, have more than one type of dementia. When this occurs, it is called mixed dementia.

Alzheimer's disease is the most common cause of dementia in people age 65 and older. It accounts for 60 to 80 percent of dementia cases.

Symptoms of dementia include:

- Having memory problems
- Repeating questions or stories over and over
- Getting lost in familiar places
- Being unable to follow directions
- Getting confused about time, people, and places
- Neglecting personal safety, hygiene, and nutrition

In addition to Alzheimer's disease, causes of dementia include depression and stroke. Both major stroke, as well as multiple small strokes can damage the brain and lead to dementia.

Dementia makes it hard to do daily tasks like driving, shopping, and visiting with friends.

9. What are the stages of Alzheimer's disease?

The National Institute on Aging and the Alzheimer's Association proposed three stages of Alzheimer's disease in their 2011 criteria and guidelines for diagnosing Alzheimer's disease.

1. Preclinical Alzheimer's disease

There are no noticeable symptoms in this stage of the disease, but changes in the brain have begun. This stage may begin up to 20 years before outward symptoms develop. Research is under way to develop tests to identify this early stage, but currently there is no established way for doctors to diagnose the disease at this stage.

2. Mild cognitive impairment due to Alzheimer's disease

During this stage of the disease, mild changes are noticeable but don't impair a person's ability to function.

3. Dementia due to Alzheimer's disease

During this stage, memory, thinking, and behavioral symptoms make it hard to function on a daily basis.

10. How long do people live with Alzheimer's disease?

The rate at which Alzheimer's disease progresses varies from person to person. In general, symptoms are mild to moderate for two to ten years and severe for the last one to five years. Most people with severe Alzheimer's disease reside in nursing homes.

The average time from diagnosis to death is eight years, but how long an individual lives with the disease varies based on age and overall health. People age 80 and older with Alzheimer's disease might live as few as three or four years, whereas younger people might live ten or more years. Still, some people live up to 20 years after they are diagnosed (see Figure 1.4).

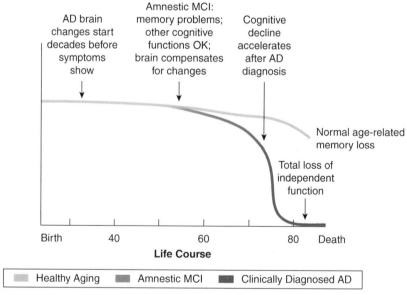

▲ **FIGURE 1.4**
Course of Alzheimer's disease.

SOURCE: Image courtesy of the National Institute on Aging/National Institutes of Health

References

1 "Alzheimer's Disease," American Academy of Neurology, accessed March 31, 2014, http://patients.aan.com/ disorders/?event=view&disorder_id=844.

2   "Understanding Alzheimer's Disease," American Academy of Neurology, 2012, accessed March 31, 2014, http://patients.aan.com/globals/axon/assets/10016.pdf.

3   "Forgetfulness: Knowing When to Ask for Help," National Institute on Aging, last updated March 11, 2014, accessed March 17, 2014, http://www.nia.nih.gov/health/publication/forgetfulness.

4   "Differences between Mild Forgetfulness and More Serious Memory Problems," National Institute on Aging, last updated March 3, 2014, accessed March 17, 2014, http://www.nia.nih.gov/alzheimers/publication/understanding-memory-loss/differences-between-mild-forgetfulness-and-more.

5   "Serious Memory Problems—Causes and Treatments," National Institute on Aging, last updated March 3, 2014, accessed March 18, 2014, http://www.nia.nih.gov/alzheimers/publication/understanding-memory-loss/serious-memory-problems-causes-and-treatments.

6   "Alzheimer's Disease Fact Sheet," National Institute on Aging, last updated December 12, 2014, accessed March 31, 2014, http://www.nia.nih.gov/alzheimers/publication/alzheimers-disease-fact-sheet.

7   "About Alzheimer's Disease: Alzheimer's Basics," National Institute on Aging, accessed March 31, 2014, http://www.nia.nih.gov/alzheimers/topics/alzheimers-basics.

8   "The Hallmarks of AD," National Institute on Aging, last updated November 14, 2014, accessed March 13, 2014, http://www.nia.nih.gov/alzheimers/publication/part-2-what-happens-brain-ad/hallmarks-ad.

9   "2014 Alzheimer's Disease Facts and Figures," Alzheimer's Association, accessed March 31, 2014, http://www.alz.org/downloads/facts_figures_2014.pdf.

10 "Inside the Brain: An Interactive Tour," Alzheimer's Association, accessed March 31, 2014, http://www.alz.org/alzheimers_disease_4719.asp.

11 "Preventing Alzheimer's Disease: What Do We Know?" National Institute on Aging, last updated January 5, 2015, accessed March 31, 2014, http://www.nia.nih.gov/alzheimers/publication/preventing-alzheimers-disease/introduction

12 "Alzheimer's & Brain Research Milestones | Research Center," Alzheimer's Association, accessed March 31, 2014, http://www.alz.org/research/science/major_milestones_in_alzheimers.asp.

13 "Emil Kraepelin (1856–1926) Psychiatric Nosographer," *JAMA* 203, no. 11 (1968): 978–9, accessed March 31, 2014, http://jama.jamanetwork.com/article.aspx?articleid=338352.

14 "Looking for the Causes of AD," National Institute on Aging, last updated March 20, 2014, accessed March 31, 2014, http://www.nia.nih.gov/alzheimers/publication/part-3-ad-research-better-questions-new-answers/looking-causes-ad.

15 Jason Karlawish, "How Are We Going to Live with Alzheimer's Disease?" *Health Affairs* 33, no. 4 (2014), 541–6, accessed May 31, 2014, http://content.healthaffairs.org/content/33/4/541.full.

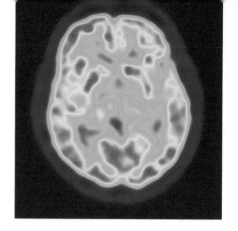

•*Causes of Alzheimer's Disease*

Case Study

Violet's daughters struggled to understand how their mother had developed Alzheimer's disease. It seemed like just yesterday that Violet was helping her granddaughter understand the complexities of algebra. What's more, Violet had always been active, strong, healthy, and sharp-minded. It just didn't make any sense.

11. What causes Alzheimer's disease?

Unfortunately, scientists don't know exactly what causes Alzheimer's disease. But research suggests that Alzheimer's disease is likely caused by a combination of your genes, your environment, and your lifestyle.

12. What factors increase the risk of Alzheimer's disease?

Like many other chronic health conditions, Alzheimer's disease develops over many years. The rare early-onset Alzheimer's disease can be caused by a genetic mutation. Most often, however, Alzheimer's disease probably develops because of several factors that are thought to increase risk.

Why Alzheimer's disease mainly strikes older adults is still unknown.

Older Age

The risk of Alzheimer's disease goes up with age. In fact, advanced age raises risk more than anything else. Most often, Alzheimer's disease is diagnosed in people age 65 and older and risk of the disease doubles every five years after age 65. Despite this, age alone cannot cause Alzheimer's disease.

Genetics

People who have a first-degree relative (parent or sibling) with Alzheimer's disease are more likely to develop the disease than people with no close family member who has had it. And those with more than one first-degree relative with the disease have an even higher the risk. Not only shared genes but shared environment or lifestyle factors may be to blame for the higher risk in family members.

Early-onset Alzheimer's disease is a rare form of Alzheimer's disease that in some cases is caused by abnormal changes (mutations) in any of three specific genes on chromosome 21, 14, or 1. The mutations play a role in generating harmful forms of amyloid plaques. If a parent caries a genetic mutation, his or her child will have a 50% chance of inheriting that mutation. If the mutation is in fact passed down, early-onset Alzheimer's disease will almost certainly develop.

In late-onset Alzheimer's disease, a single gene on chromosome 19 called apolipoprotein E (APOE) has been linked with risk of late-onset Alzheimer's disease. There are three forms of the gene—e2, e3, and e4—and you inherit one of the three forms from each parent. The e4 form, which not many people in the United States have, is thought to increase the risk of Alzheimer's disease.

Scientists have identified a number of other genes that might increase the risk of late-onset Alzheimer's disease and continue to look for more.

Factors that Cause Heart Disease

Smoking, obesity, diabetes, high cholesterol in midlife, and high blood pressure in midlife are linked with a higher risk of Alzheimer's disease. They also increase the risk of heart disease. Research suggests that the health of the brain depends on the health of the heart and blood vessels.

Less Education

People who have fewer years of school have a higher risk of Alzheimer's disease. Some experts think this is because having more years of formal education might increase the number of connections between nerve cells in the brain, which might help create alternative routes of communication between nerve cells when Alzheimer's disease starts to damage the brain.

Race

Older African-American and Hispanic people are more likely than older white people to develop Alzheimer's disease. The

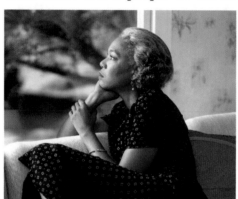

risk is two times higher for African-Americans and one and a half times higher for Hispanics. Higher rates of diabetes and high blood pressure, as well as lower average levels of education, are thought to account for the higher Alzheimer's disease rates in these populations.

Brain Injury

A head injury, like a blow or jolt to the head, that upsets normal brain function is called a traumatic brain injury (TBI). A moderate or severe TBI increases risk for Alzheimer's disease.

Table 2.1 Traumatic Brain Injury and Risk of Alzheimer's Disease

TBI SEVERITY	SYMPTOMS	RISK OF ALZHEIMER'S DISEASE (COMPARED WITH NO HEAD INJURY)
Moderate	Loss of consciousness or amnesia for at least 30 minutes	Two times as high
Severe	Loss of consciousness or amnesia for more than 24 hours	More than four times as high

SOURCE: Alzheimer's Association, 2014 Alzheimer's Disease Facts and Figures, *Alzheimer's & Dementia*, Volume 10, Issue 2.

Other factors may also play a role in increasing risk for Alzheimer's disease, including having low numbers of red blood cells (anemia).

Early-onset Alzheimer's disease can be inherited. This rare form of Alzheimer's disease can be caused by abnormal changes (mutations) that are passed down in any of three specific genes, called:

- amyloid precursor protein gene
- presenilin 1 protein gene
- presenilin 2 protein gene

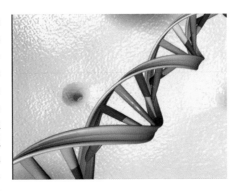

One percent or fewer people with Alzheimer's disease have these mutations, but inheriting them nearly guarantees that a person will develop the disease. For most of these people, symptoms will begin before age 65, but some will develop signs of the disease as early as age 30. Genetic testing is available for people with a family history of early-onset Alzheimer's disease.

The more common late-onset Alzheimer's disease has been linked with a gene called apolipoprotein E (APOE). There are three common forms of the gene—e2, e3, and e4—and you inherit one of the three forms from each parent.

Table 2.2 APOE Gene and Risk for Alzheimer's Disease

INHERITED APOE FORMS	PERCENTAGE OF PEOPLE IN U.S. WITH EACH FORM	EFFECT ON RISK OF ALZHEIMER'S DISEASE
Two copies of APOE-e3	60 percent	No effect
One or two copies of APOE-e4	20–30 percent	Somewhat increases risk
One or two copies of APOE-e2	10–20 percent	May decrease risk
Two copies of APOE-e4	2 percent	Increases risk most

SOURCE: Alzheimer's Association, 2014 Alzheimer's Disease Facts and Figures, *Alzheimer's & Dementia*, Volume 10, Issue 2.

About 40 percent of people with late-onset Alzheimer's disease have one or two copies of the APOE-e4 gene. But unlike the three known gene *mutations* that actually *cause* changes in the brain that lead to early-onset Alzheimer's disease, having one or two copies of the APOE-e4 gene increases only the *risk* of the disease. Likewise, people with other forms of the APOE gene can also develop the disease.

For a video on Alzheimer's disease and genetics, visit

http://www.alz.org/research/science/alzheimers_disease_causes.asp

ON THE WEB

To learn more about genetics, see the "Alzheimer's Disease Genetics Fact Sheet."

ON THE CD

Genetic testing for APOE gene forms cannot predict who will develop Alzheimer's disease and is currently used only in research settings. It is unlikely to ever forecast who will get the disease with 100 percent accuracy because so many factors influence risk.

A number of other genes have also been linked with late-onset Alzheimer's disease.

14. Can Alzheimer's disease be prevented?

There is no clear answer for how to prevent Alzheimer's disease. But several healthy lifestyle factors have been linked with lower risk.

Physical Activity

Exercise and staying physically active is essential to good health. Regular physical activity strengthens muscles, improves heart and lung function, helps prevent osteoporosis (bone weakness), and boosts mood and overall well-being. Some studies suggest that it may also play a role in lowering risk for Alzheimer's disease. One study, for example, found that older adults who took part in a brisk walking program for six months had increased nerve cell activity in key parts of

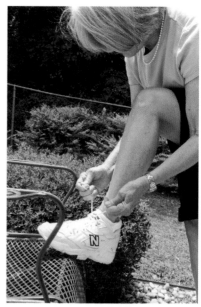

the brain. Being active might help the brain maintain older connections between brain cells and create new ones, too.

Heart-Healthy Diet

Research suggests that what you eat may influence risk of Alzheimer's disease. For example, two studies found that people who ate the most vegetables, especially green leafy vegetables and cruciferous ones like broccoli, had a slower rate of cognitive decline than those who ate the least of these foods. Another study found that those who ate a "Mediterranean diet" had a lower risk of Alzheimer's disease.

Features of a Mediterranean diet include:

- High amounts of vegetables, fruits, legumes (such as beans and lentils), and cereals
- Low to moderate amounts of dairy products, fish, and poultry
- Low to moderate amounts of wine
- Low amounts of red meat
- Frequent use of olive oil

For more information on a Mediterranean diet read "Welcome to the Mediterranean Diet."

Mental and Social Activity

Staying social and keeping your mind active may help lower your risk of Alzheimer's disease. Large studies in older people have shown that those who were the most social or took part

You can stay socially engaged through work, volunteering, or living with someone.

Activities such as reading books, magazines, and newspapers; going to lectures; listening to the radio; visiting museums; and playing games can help you stay cognitively active.

To keep chronic diseases at bay and improve your overall health, follow these tips:

- Exercise on a regular basis
- Eat a healthy diet with lots of fruits and vegetables
- Stay socially active
- Engage in activities that stimulate your mind
- Prevent or control type 2 diabetes
- Prevent or lower high blood pressure levels
- Prevent or lower high cholesterol levels
- Keep or work towards a healthy weight
- Don't smoke, or quit smoking

◀ FIGURE 2.1
Healthy Body, Healthy Brain

Many other approaches are being studied to see if they might help prevent Alzheimer's disease, including a possible vaccine. To learn more about preventing Alzheimer's disease, including what research is under way, see "Preventing Alzheimer's Disease: What Do We Know?" at

http://www.nia.nih.gov/sites/default/files/preventing_alzheimers_disease_0.pdf

ON THE CD

in activities that were intellectually engaging had a lower risk of Alzheimer's disease.

There is some evidence that formal cognitive training, such as memory training, reasoning training, or processing-speed training, improves mental skills, even 10 years after the training is completed.

15. Do any vitamins or dietary supplements help prevent Alzheimer's disease?

Researchers have looked at whether a number of vitamins and dietary supplements can help protect the brain from Alzheimer's disease. But the evidence is mixed, so the jury is still out. Here's what the research has shown so far.

DHA

Studies in mice showed that an omega-3 fatty acid found in salmon and other fish, called docosahexaenoic acid (DHA), reduced the number of harmful Alzheimer's plaques in the brain. However, DHA showed no effect in a study of people with mild to moderate disease. It is possible, however, that DHA supplements might be helpful if taken before Alzheimer's symptoms begin.

Antioxidants

Some research suggests that antioxidants—such as vitamins E, C, and B; ginkgo biloba; and coenzyme Q—in food or dietary supplements may lower the risk of Alzheimer's disease. But clinical trials in humans have found no effect.

Resveratrol

Studies in animals have found that a compound found in red grapes called resveratrol can reduce the number of Alzheimer's plaques in the brain. Studies in humans have shown that people who drink a moderate amount of red wine have a lower risk of developing

Talk with a doctor before using any vitamins or supplements that claim to help prevent or treat Alzheimer's disease.

NOTE

Alzheimer's disease. A clinical study is under way to test the effect of resveratrol in people with Alzheimer's disease.

ON THE WEB

For more information about vitamins and dietary supplements, visit the National Center for Complementary and Integrative Health at

https://nccih.nih.gov.

REFERENCE

References

1   "Alzheimer's Disease Fact Sheet," National Institute on Aging, last updated December 12, 2014, accessed March 31, 2014, http://www.nia .nih.gov/alzheimers/publication/alzheimers-disease-fact-sheet.

2   "2014 Alzheimer's Disease Facts and Figures," Alzheimer's Association, accessed March 31, 2014, http://www.alz.org/downloads/facts_ figures_2014.pdf.

3   "About Alzheimer's Disease: Causes," National Institute on Aging, accessed March 31, 2014, http://www.nia.nih.gov/alzheimers/topics/ causes.

4   "Alzheimer's Disease," American Academy of Neurology, accessed March 31, 2014, http://patients.aan.com/ disorders/?event=view&disorder_id=844.

5   "Preventing Alzheimer's Disease: What Do We Know?" National Institute on Aging, last updated January 5, 2015, accessed March 31, 2014, http://www.nia.nih.gov/alzheimers/publication/preventing-alzheimers-disease/introduction.

6   "Looking for the Causes of AD," National Institute on Aging, last updated March 20, 2014, accessed March 31, 2014, http://www.nia.nih .gov/alzheimers/publication/part-3-ad-research-better-questions-new-answers/looking-causes-ad.

7   "Younger/Early Onset | Alzheimer's Association," Alzheimer's Association, accessed March 31, 2014, http://www.alz.org/alzheimers_ disease_early_onset.asp.

8   "Alzheimer's Disease Genetics Fact Sheet," National Institute on Aging, June 2011, accessed March 31, 2014, http://www.nia.nih.gov/ sites/default/files/alzheimers_disease_genetics_fact_sheet_1.pdf.

9   Chang Hyung Hong et al, "Anemia and Risk of Dementia in Older Adults: Findings from the Health ABC Study." *Neurology* 81, no. 6 (2013), 528–33. doi:10.1212/WNL.0b013e31829e701d.

10   "Looking for the Causes of AD," National Institute on Aging, last updated March 20, 2014, accessed March 31, 2014, http://www.nia.nih .gov/alzheimers/publication/part-3-ad-research-better-questions-new-answers/looking-causes-ad.

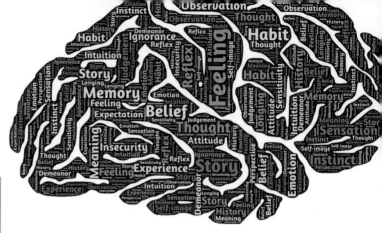

•*Alzheimer's Disease Symptoms*

Case Study

Like most people with Alzheimer's disease, Violet started having mild symptoms that worsened over time. Looking back, one of the first symptoms that her family noticed was that she had a hard time deciding what to order when they went out to eat. Her daughters would encourage her to start looking at the menu right away. They would tease, "Mom, no talking; only looking."

Writing notes on scraps of paper to compensate for her failing memory followed. The notes became increasingly disorganized and eventually were written on the walls. Violet knew something was wrong and confided in a neighbor, but she didn't share her worries with her children, who were becoming increasingly concerned too.

After her diagnosis, as the disease progressed, Violet began gardening at midnight, getting lost going to familiar places, and hoarding. But there were still many good days that she and her daughters enjoyed and made the most of.

Today, Violet's symptoms are typical of severe Alzheimer's disease. Unable to sit up in her wheelchair, she now spends her days in bed. But she sometimes makes eye contact with her daughters and can still respond to questions with a "yes" or "no."

16. What are the symptoms of mild Alzheimer's disease?

The rate at which Alzheimer's disease progresses from mild to moderate to severe differs in different people. Knowing what to expect in general as the disease progresses can help you plan ahead.

Experts think that the disease actually begins to damage the brain 20 or more years before symptoms become noticeable.

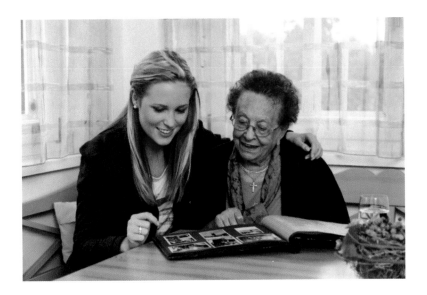

This period of time is sometimes called the preclinical stage of Alzheimer's disease.

As damage to the brain increases, however, symptoms of mild disease eventually develop; these can include:

- Memory loss
- Confusion about the locations of familiar places
- Taking longer than normal to do daily tasks
- Difficulty handling money and paying bills
- Poor judgment that leads to bad choices
- Loss of spontaneity and initiative
- Mood and personality changes, including more anxiety and aggression

People with mild Alzheimer's disease may be healthy otherwise and can still make meaningful contributions to their family and society. They can also take part in decisions about their care.

For example, a person with mild Alzheimer's symptoms might ask the same question over and over throughout the day or often misplace items like their glasses or keys.

17. What are the symptoms of moderate Alzheimer's disease?

In moderate Alzheimer's disease, damage has spread into the areas of the brain that control language, reasoning, sensory processing, and conscious thought. As a result, symptoms become more noticeable and frequent. They can include:

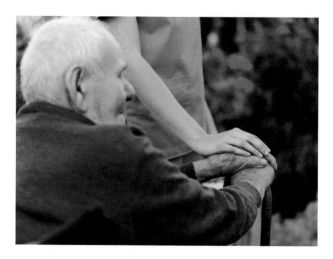

- Increasing memory loss and confusion
- Shortened attention span
- Inappropriate anger
- Trouble recognizing loved ones
- Difficulty thinking logically
- Inability to learn new things
- Difficulty coping with new or unexpected situations
- Restlessness, agitation, anxiety, tearfulness, wandering (especially in the late afternoon or night)
- Hallucinations, delusions, suspiciousness or paranoia, irritability
- Inability to do tasks with multiple steps, like setting the table or getting dressed

Despite these symptoms, people with moderate Alzheimer's disease may still enjoy normal activities.

For example, they may no longer be able to do complex tasks like drive a car safely or use public transportation.

18. What are the symptoms of severe Alzheimer's disease?

In severe Alzheimer's disease, damage to the brain is widespread. People with severe Alzheimer's disease are totally dependent on others for care. They can no longer recognize people they know or communicate in any way. They are often in bed most or all of the time.

People with severe Alzheimer's disease may need to move to a residential care facility for around-the-clock care.

In this final stage of the disease, people need help with activities of daily living, including bathing, dressing, eating, and using the bathroom. Other symptoms can include:

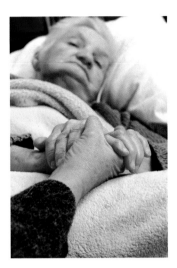

- Weight loss
- Seizures
- Skin infections
- Trouble swallowing
- Groaning, moaning, or grunting
- Increased sleeping
- Lack of bladder and bowel control

19. Is depression linked with Alzheimer's disease?

Nearly half of people with Alzheimer's disease also have depression. It is especially common in people with mild or moderate Alzheimer's disease.

Many people become depressed when they realize that their memory and ability to function are getting worse.

It can be hard to tell if someone with Alzheimer's disease also has depression, though. This is because the person may not be able to express his or her feelings and because dementia and depression can cause some of the same symptoms, such as:

- Apathy
- Social withdrawal
- Isolation
- Difficulty concentrating
- Impaired thinking
- Loss of interest in activities and hobbies

The good news is that treatment for depression can boost quality of life and function. If you think depression is present, ask your doctor for a referral to see a geriatric psychiatrist.

A geriatric psychiatrist is a doctor who specializes in recognizing and treating depression and other mental disorders in older people.

A person with Alzheimer's disease is considered to have depression if he or she has a depressed mood (sad, hopeless, discouraged, or

Telling someone with depression to "cheer up" or "try harder" isn't helpful. Instead, the person needs support, reassurance, and help from a mental health professional.

To learn more about depression and Alzheimer's disease, visit

https://www.alz.org/care/alzheimers-dementia-depression.asp.

tearful), less pleasure from usual activities, and two of the following:

- Social isolation or withdrawal
- Changes in appetite that are not caused by another health problem
- Changes in sleep patterns
- Agitation or slowed speech and movements
- Irritability
- Fatigue or low energy
- Feelings of worthlessness or hopelessness, or inappropriate or excessive guilt
- Thoughts of death, suicide plans, or a suicide attempt

Most people with Alzheimer's disease and depression are treated with medicine, talk therapy, and a gradual return to activities they enjoy.

20. What behavioral symptoms occur in Alzheimer's disease?

Although Alzheimer's disease is often thought of as a **cognitive disorder** that affects memory, language, thinking, and reasoning, most people with Alzheimer's disease also experience **behavioral** and **psychiatric** symptoms at some point. These symptoms are called **neuropsychiatric** symptoms because they are psychiatric symptoms caused by a brain disorder.

Behavioral and psychiatric symptoms can be among the most challenging and distressing effects of the disease. In fact, they often carry the most weight in deciding whether a person needs to be placed in a residential care program.

Behavioral and psychiatric symptoms can include:

- Personality changes, such as irritability, anxiety, apathy, or depression
- Sleep problems
- **Agitation**, such as physical or verbal outbursts, general emotional distress, restlessness, pacing, shredding paper or tissues, or yelling

- Delusions, which are firmly held beliefs in things that are not real
- Hallucinations, which means seeing, hearing, or feeling things that are not there.

Apathy is a disorder of motivation in which a person lacks goal-oriented behavior, cognition, or emotion. A lack of interest is one of the core features.

Depression and apathy are the most common neuropsychiatric symptoms in Alzheimer's disease.

21. What other medical problems are linked with Alzheimer's disease?

People with Alzheimer's disease have a higher risk of seizures. Up to one out of five patients with Alzheimer's disease experience them, especially during the early stages of the disease. Cognitive decline tends to begin sooner in patients with Alzheimer's disease who have seizures.

Signs of seizures in people with Alzheimer's disease include:

- Passing problems with speaking, listening, reading, or writing (aphasia)
- Periods of memory loss (amnestic spells)
- Having Déjà vu

Various medications, including levetiracetam and lamotrigine, appear effective at suppressing seizures in people with Alzheimer's disease.

In addition, people with Alzheimer's disease have higher rates of various health problems, especially vascular disease, than those without Alzheimer's disease. These problems include:

- Heart disease
- Stroke
- Diabetes
- High blood pressure
- Sleep apnea (disorder that causes breathing pauses during sleep)
- Osteoporosis (bone weakness)
- Glaucoma (disease that damages the eye's optic nerve)

Many people with Alzheimer's disease also experience other types of health problems. Because of this, they will need health care to deal with more than the behavioral and psychological symptoms of the disease.

22. When should a doctor be contacted about symptoms?

Many people are unsure when to see a doctor about forgetfulness or other behavior problems. That's because it can be hard to know when memory problems are a sign of something serious or just a normal part of aging. You don't have to sort this out yourself, however. The time to see a doctor is when you are worried about memory problems or any other symptoms.

When you see a doctor, Sharing the symptoms you are experiencing is one of the most important things you can do to help you doctor make a diagnosis or track the progress of your disease.

✓ Give a basic one- or two-sentence description of your problems.

✓ Explain when the symptoms occur and how often they occur.

✓ Describe what makes the symptoms better or worse.

✓ Mention whether you have had the symptoms before and under what circumstances.

✓ Say whether other family members have had the same symptoms.

▲ **FIGURE 3.1**
How to tell your doctor about your symptoms.

For more information about how to talk with your doctor, read *Talking with Your Doctor – A Guide for Older People* from the National Institute on Aging.

ON THE CD

Before you leave your doctor's office, make a follow-up appointment for sometime in the next 6 to 12 months to check your memory.

23. How does someone die from Alzheimer's disease?

The cause of death for most people with Alzheimer's disease is aspiration pneumonia. This can occur during severe dementia when a person is unable to swallow properly and takes food or liquid into the lungs instead of into the stomach. In cases like this, pneumonia, instead of dementia, may be listed as the immediate cause of death.

Regardless of the offi cial cause of death, Researchers estimate that among 70-year-olds, those with Alzheimer's disease are more likely to die before they turn 80 than those without the disease (61% versus 30%, respectively).

NOTE

The average time from diagnosis of Alzheimer's dementia to death is three to nine years.

1   "2014 Alzheimer's Disease Facts and Figures," Alzheimer's Association, accessed March 31, 2014, http://www.alz.org/downloads/facts_figures_2014.pdf,.

2   "Alzheimer's Disease Fact Sheet," National Institute on Aging, last updated December 12, 2014, accessed March 31, 2014, http://www.nia.nih.gov/alzheimers/publication/alzheimers-disease-fact-sheet.

3   "Forgetfulness: Knowing When to Ask for Help," National Institute on Aging, last updated March 11, 2014, accessed March 31, 2014, http://www.nia.nih.gov/health/publication/forgetfulness.

4   "Alzheimer's Disease: Unraveling the Mystery," National Institute on Aging, last updated March 20, 2014, accessed March 31, 2014, http://www.nia.nih.gov/alzheimers/publication/part-2-what-happens-brain-ad/changing-brain-ad.

5   Jason Karlawish, "How Are We Going to Live with Alzheimer's Disease?" *Health Affairs* 33, no. 4 (2014), 541–46, accessed May 31, 2014, http://content.healthaffairs.org/content/33/4/541.full.

6   "Alzheimer's Stages and Changes, U.S. Department of Health and Human Services, accessed May 31, 2014, http://www.alzheimers.gov/alzheimers_stages.html.

7   "Depression and Alzheimer's Disease," American Academy of Family Physicians, accessed May 31, 2014, http://familydoctor.org/familydoctor/en/diseases-conditions/dementia/complications/depression-and-alzheimers-disease.html.

8   "Depression and Alzheimer's," Alzheimer's Association, accessed May 31, 2014, http://www.alz.org/care/alzheimers-dementia-depression.asp.

9   Constantine G. Lyketsos et al., "Neuropsychiatric Symptoms in Alzheimer's Disease." *Alzheimer's & Dementia: The Journal of the Alzheimer's Association* 7, no. 5 (2011), 532–39. www.alzheimersanddementia.com/article/S1552-5260(11)02575-1/abstract.

10 "Behavioral Symptoms," Alzheimer's Association, accessed May 31, 2014, available at http://www.alz.org/professionals_and_researchers_behavioral_symptoms_pr.asp.

11 Michel Benoit et al., "Apathy and Depression in Mild Alzheimer's Disease: A Cross-Sectional Study Using Diagnostic Criteria." *Journal of Alzheimer's Disease* 31, no. 2 (2012), 325–34.

12 Keith A. Vossel et al., "Seizures and Epileptiform Activity in the Early Stages of Alzheimer Disease," *JAMA Neurology* 70, no. 9 (2013), 1158–66. doi:10.1001/jamaneurol.2013.136.

13 A. Duthie et al, "Non-Psychiatric Comorbidity Associated with Alzheimer's Disease," *QJM* 104, no. 11 (2011), 913–20. doi:10.1093/qjmed/hcr118.

14 Fred Andersen et al., "Co-Morbidity and Drug Treatment in Alzheimer's Disease. A Cross Sectional Study of Participants in the Dementia Study in Northern Norway," *BMC Geriatrics* 11, no. 58 (2011), www.ncbi.nlm.nih.gov/pmc/articles/PMC3204237/.

15 "Talking About Symptoms With Your Health Care Team," Center for Advancing Health, accessed May 31, 2014, http://www.cfah.org/prepared-patient/prepared-patient-articles/talking-about-symptoms-with-your-health-care-team#.UQ09O2dLp8E?utm_source=CFAH+Digest+4.9.14&utm_campaign=CFAH+Digest+4.9.14&utm_medium=email.

16 Bryan. D. James et al, "Contribution of Alzheimer Disease to Mortality in the United States," *Neurology* 82:12 (2014), 1045–50. www.neurology.org/content/82/12/1045.

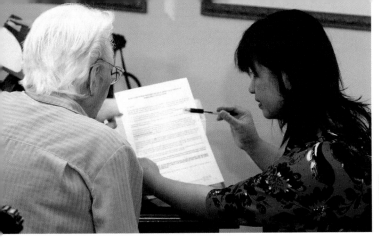

Diagnosis of Alzheimer's Disease •

Before Alzheimer's disease symptoms developed, cancer and stroke were the health problems Violet worried about the most. Because she had a family history of cancer and stroke she was vigilant in looking for signs of either of them, and so were her daughters. So when Violet's increasingly troubling behavior prompted her daughters to take her to her primary care doctor, they were stunned to hear that he thought she had Alzheimer's disease.

After an initial brief screening assessment that included asking Violet to spell "apple" and name the current month, her primary care doctor referred her to a psychiatrist for a complete evaluation.

The psychiatrist performed additional tests and talked with Violet and her two daughters who accompanied her about her symptoms and behavior—including that she had been repeatedly purchasing the same item though mail-order shopping. The evaluation confirmed the primary care doctor's suspicion that Violet had Alzheimer's disease.

Violet was not bothered by her diagnosis; an effect of her disease. But her daughters felt blindsided and unprepared.

24. How is Alzheimer's disease diagnosed?

Most often, people go to their primary care doctor when concerns about memory or behavior arise, and Alzheimer's disease is usually diagnosed when the symptoms are still mild.

There are a number of steps that doctors take to evaluate a person for Alzheimer's disease. They usually include a general exam and an assessment of cognitive function (such as attention and memory), daily function (such as the ability to cook, shop, and manage finances), and behavior problems (such as anxiety and apathy).

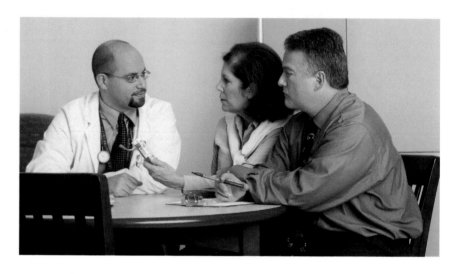

General exam

First, a doctor will look for coexisting health problems, factors that increase the risk of Alzheimer's disease, and other possible causes of cognitive impairment. To do this, your doctor may:

- Review your medical history (see Figure 4.1)
- Conduct a physical exam
- Review your medicines, both over-the-counter and prescription
- Test your blood and urine
- Refer you for a brain scan, if necessary
- Ask for input from family members

Your doctor will ask you questions about your medical and family history, including any prior mental health problems, cognitive changes, and behavior changes. He or she may also ask:

- Have you had any recent illnesses?
- Have you used any new prescription or over-the-counter medications that could cause memory loss, such as benzodiazepines for trouble sleeping or anticholinergic drugs for urinary incontinence?
- Have you used or been exposed to illicit drugs?
- Have you been exposed to environmental toxins, such as fuels or solvents?
- Have you had any recent head injuries?
- Do you have any history of seizures?

▲ FIGURE 4.1
Common Questions During the Medical History

Assessment of cognitive function, daily function, and behavior problems

There are various tests that can be used to evaluate cognitive performance, level of independence, and severity of behavioral symptoms. Most take only a few minutes to complete. Some are completed by the patient, others by someone close to the patient. These tests also provide a snapshot of cognitive ability that can be used as a baseline to compare with abilities in the future.

Based on the results of the general exam and tests of cognitive ability, your doctor will determine if you have mild cognitive impairment or dementia (see Tables 4.1 and 4.2).

Table 4.1 Core Criteria for Mild Cognitive Impairment (MCI)

DIAGNOSIS OF MCI REQUIRES:
• Concern about a change in cognition relative to previous functioning
• Lower performance than expected for the person's age and education in one or more cognitive functions, like memory and problem solving, ideally based on cognitive tests (Memory is the function most commonly impaired in people who go from MCI to Alzheimer's dementia.)
• Preserved ability to function independently in daily life, though some complex tasks such as paying bills or shopping may be more difficult than before
• No evidence of substantial impairment; no dementia

SOURCE: Marilyn S. Albert et al., "The Diagnosis of Mild Cognitive Impairment due to Alzheimer's Disease: Recommendations from the National Institute on Aging-Alzheimer's Association Workgroups on Diagnostic Guidelines for Alzheimer's Disease." *Alzheimer's & Dementia* 7, no. 3 (2011), 270–9.

Table 4.2 Core Criteria for Dementia

DIAGNOSIS OF DEMENTIA REQUIRES:
1. Cognitive or behavioral symptoms that • Interfere with the ability to function at work or during usual activities, • Are worse than before, and • Cannot be explained by delirium or a mental health disorder.
2. Detection of cognitive or behavioral symptoms through discussion with the patient and caregiver and through some form of testing
3. Cognitive or behavioral impairment involving at least two of the following "domains" • Impaired ability to acquire and remember new information (such as repeating questions or conversations) • Impaired reasoning and handling of complex tasks, poor judgment (such as inability to manage finances) • Impaired visual/spatial abilities (such as being unable to find objects in direct view) • Impaired speaking, reading, or writing abilities (such as trouble thinking of common words when talking) • Changes in personality or behavior (such as agitation or apathy)

SOURCE: Guy M. McKhann et al., "The Diagnosis of Dementia due to Alzheimer's Disease: Recommendations from the National Institute on Aging-Alzheimer's Association Workgroups on Diagnostic Guidelines for Alzheimer's Disease." *Alzheimer's & Dementia* 7, no. 3 (2011), 263–9.

Finally, for dementia to be considered to result from Alzheimer's disease, it must also have these characteristics:

- gradual onset of symptoms over months to years (not over hours or days),
- clear worsening of cognition according to report or observation
- cognitive problems evident in the person's history and examination in the first four domains in Table 4.2
- no evidence of another health problem that is affecting cognition

The diagnosis is considered probable Alzheimer's disease dementia if the patient meets the criteria for dementia and also has these additional characteristics. The diagnosis is considered possible Alzheimer's disease dementia if the patient doesn't meet all the criteria for Alzheimer's disease dementia or there is evidence that other conditions are present that may also affect cognition.

To learn more about diagnosing Alzheimer's disease, watch the video *Diagnosing Alzheimer's Disease* from the National Institutes of Health at

http://nihseniorhealth.gov/videolist.html#alzheimersdisease

25. Will I be referred to a specialist for diagnosis?

Many primary care doctors can diagnose Alzheimer's disease. However, if your primary care doctor is uncertain that Alzheimer's disease is the cause of your symptoms, he or she may refer you to a specialist for additional evaluation. Specialists who diagnose Alzheimer's disease include:

- geriatricians, who manage health care in older adults and specialize in how the body changes as it ages
- neurologists, who specialize in the health of the brain and can carry out and review brain scans
- psychiatrists, who specialize in mental and emotional health
- geriatric psychiatrists, who specialize in the mental and emotional health of older adults
- neuropsychologists, who conduct tests of memory and thinking

Some people choose to see a specialist on their own. You can find specialists through memory clinics and centers or through local organizations or referral services.

26. What other health problems can cause memory trouble?

Dementia and memory problems can be caused by many factors other than Alzheimer's disease. Memory problems can be caused by a number of health issues, including:

- Medication side effects
- Low levels of vitamin B12
- Alcohol abuse
- Brain tumors
- Infection in the brain
- Blood clots in the brain
- Certain thyroid, kidney, or liver problems

These are serious medical conditions that should be treated right away.

Stress, anxiety, and depression can also leave you more forgetful or confused. These feelings can arise from many circumstances, including coping with major life changes like losing a loved one or retiring. But the confusion and forgetfulness go away as the strong feelings fade.

In addition, the combination of high blood pressure, high cholesterol, and diabetes can cause confusion and problems with memory.

27. Is a brain scan needed to diagnose Alzheimer's disease?

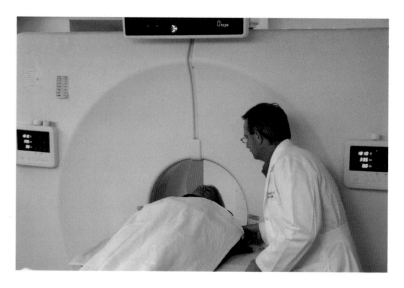

Even after a thorough medical exam, it's not always clear what is causing dementia. A magnetic resonance imaging (MRI) scan or a computed tomography (CT) scan may be ordered to help rule out certain causes of dementia, such as a stroke or trauma to the head. Both types of scans make a cross-sectional picture of your brain. An MRI uses magnetic fields and a computer, and a CT uses X-rays and a computer.

If the cause of dementia is still unknown, a positron emission tomography (PET) scan may help diagnose the problem. A PET scan uses a radioactive substance, which is injected through a vein, to show on a computer monitor how the brain is working.

When used along with a radioactive drug, a PET scan can show if you have the telltale plaques of Alzheimer's disease. If the scan shows that you don't have plaques, then it is much less likely that you have Alzheimer's disease.

Because PET scans emit small amounts of radiation and are expensive (and typically not covered by insurance), only those with serious memory loss with no known cause after a complete evaluation should receive this scan.

28. What are Alzheimer's disease biomarkers?

According to the Alzheimer's Association, a biomarker is a "biological factor that can be measured to indicate the presence or absence of a disease, or the risk for developing a disease."

Examples of biomarkers include blood sugar level as an indicator of diabetes and cholesterol as an indicator of heart disease risk.

Biomarkers for Alzheimer's disease are being researched as a potential way to help to detect onset of the disease before symptoms are noticeable, as well as to track disease progression. Researchers think that future treatments for Alzheimer's disease will be most effective when started in the preclinical stage, which biomarkers will be able to identify. Biomarkers may also help indicate if treatment is effective.

There are currently two main types of biomarkers for Alzheimer's disease: those that measure the amount of beta-amyloid in the brain and those that measure neuron damage.

Levels of beta-amyloid and tau in cerebrospinal fluid and blood are being studied as potential biomarkers of the disease, but they are used only in the research setting right now.

Because biomarkers are still under research, diagnosis of Alzheimer's disease still depends on assessing cognition and function.

29. Who should attend Alzheimer's disease testing and diagnosis?

It's important for the person being evaluated to bring along a family member or close friend who can provide input and help answer the doctor's questions. It is by discussing the daily affairs and functioning of the patient with both the patient and a knowledgeable person close to him or her that a doctor can make an informed diagnosis.

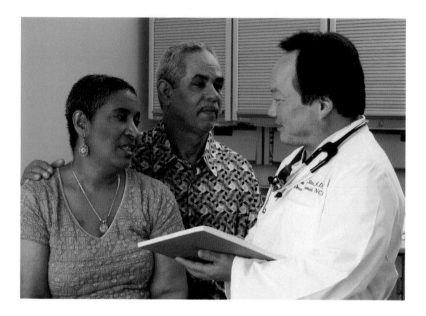

As part of the evaluation of Alzheimer's disease, the doctor may want to identify who will be the main caregiver. The primary caregiver is an essential member of the health care team of someone with Alzheimer's disease.

In fact, the doctor may also check on the physical and emotional health of the caregiver over time. That's because the health of a caregiver is essential to that of a person with Alzheimer's disease. In addition to providing resources for the caregiver, the doctor may refer him or her to other health care providers and services for additional support.

30. What are the Alzheimer's diagnostic guidelines?

Proposed revised criteria and guidelines for the diagnosis of Alzheimer's disease were published in 2011 by expert panels brought together by the National Institute on Aging and the Alzheimer's Association. These updated guidelines reflect advances in the understanding of the disease. The original guidelines, which were published in 1984, defined Alzheimer's disease as having only one stage, dementia. Diagnosis was based solely on symptoms, too.

The new guidelines reflect current understanding of the disease, mainly that there are three distinct stages: the preclinical stage, mild cognitive impairment (MCI), and Alzheimer's dementia.

In addition, the guidelines address the use of imaging and biomarkers in blood and spinal fluid. These technologies may help determine if changes in the brain and body fluid are due to Alzheimer's disease.

The new guidelines also make a distinction between *changes* in the brain and actual *symptoms* of the disease.

To learn more about the new Guidelines, read *Diagnostic Guidelines for Alzheimer's Disease: Frequently Asked Questions for the General Public* from the National Institute on Aging's Alzheimer's Disease Education and Referral Center. Search for "diagnostic guidelines frequently asked questions" at

http://www.nia.nih.gov/alzheimers.

31. What are the benefits of early diagnosis?

It is better for both patients and their families to find out sooner rather than later if they have Alzheimer's disease. With an early diagnosis, people with the disease can still participate in planning their care and preparing for future challenges, by:

- making living arrangements
- taking care of financial and legal matters
- developing support networks

In addition, treatment is most likely to provide benefit when it is started early, and an early diagnosis can provide more opportunities for people with Alzheimer's disease to volunteer for clinical trials and develop strong relationships with doctors and caregivers.

32. What types of doctors can diagnose Alzheimer's disease?

Most often, Alzheimer's disease is diagnosed by a person's primary care doctor. But specialists diagnose the disease too, including:

- geriatricians
- neurologists
- psychiatrists

- geriatric psychiatrists
- neuropsychologists

33. What are memory centers?

Memory clinics, or memory centers, have teams of specialists who work together to diagnose Alzheimer's disease. Tests are done at the clinic or center, which can speed the time to diagnosis.

34. What are Alzheimer's Disease Research Centers?

Alzheimer's Disease Research Centers are major medical institutions in the United States that receive funding from the National Institute on Aging to translate research advances into better diagnosis and care for Alzheimer's disease. These centers are also working to find ways to cure or prevent Alzheimer's disease.

To find the Alzheimer's Disease Research Center nearest you, visit

http://www.nia.nih.gov/alzheimers/alzheimers-disease-research-centers.

ON THE WEB

In addition to conducting research, Alzheimer's Disease Research Centers offer services to people with Alzheimer's disease and their caregivers, including:

- help with Alzheimer's disease diagnosis and management
- information about the disease and about services and resources for people who have it
- opportunities to participate in clinical trials, support groups, clinical research projects, and other special programs

35. Should I get a second opinion?

Diagnosis of memory and thinking problems can be a challenge because the signs and symptoms of Alzheimer's disease can be subtle or unclear. Most doctors understand the benefit of getting a second opinion and will share your records with another doctor if you sign a form permitting them to. You can ask your doctor for a referral to a specialist for a second opinion, or you can look for a specialist yourself. You can find specialists through memory clinics and centers or through local organizations or referral services.

It is normal to be unsure about what to ask after being diagnosed with Alzheimer's disease. You need some time to process the news.

If you find yourself ready to learn a bit about the disease, however, consider asking these questions:

- How did you come to decide that I have Alzheimer's disease?
- How will the disease progress?
- What can I expect in the future?
- What resources exist to help my family and me learn more about the disease?
- Will you manage my future care?

In addition, when you are being evaluated for Alzheimer's disease, you have the right to a dignified experience. "Principles for a Dignified Diagnosis" from the Alzheimer's Association was written by people with dementia to help set standards for what to expect during the process of being diagnosed with Alzheimer's disease (see Figure 4.2).

For a comprehensive list of questions for your doctor, read *Questions for Your Doctor* from the Alzheimer's Association.

Read more about each of the "Principles for a Dignified Diagnosis."

✓ Talk to me directly, the person with dementia.
✓ Tell the truth.
✓ Test early.
✓ Take my concerns seriously, regardless of my age.
✓ Deliver the news in plain but sensitive language.
✓ Coordinate with other care providers.
✓ Explain the purpose of different tests and what you hope to learn.
✓ Give me tools for living with this disease.
✓ Work with me on a plan for healthy living.
✓ Recognize that I am an individual and the way I experience this disease is unique.
✓ Alzheimer's is a journey, not a destination.

▲ FIGURE 4.2
Alzheimer's Association's Principles for a Dignified Diagnosis.

37. How can I cope with the diagnosis?

Being diagnosed with Alzheimer's disease is a life-changing event. It is normal to have a range of emotions, including anger, relief, denial, depression, resentment, fear, isolation, and loss.

Try to find healthy ways to deal with these emotions. The Alzheimer's Association recommends these approaches:

- Share how you feel with friends and loved ones.
- Talk with a counselor or clergyperson.
- Write down your thoughts in a journal.
- Keep up your social activities, hobbies, and creative interests.

Depression and anxiety are common emotions that everyone feels once in a while. When they don't go away or are strong enough to disturb your daily life, they could be signs of a depressive or anxiety disorder. Both types of disorders can be treated so that you can accept your diagnosis, move ahead, and find ways to live fully.

For more information on what to do after a diagnosis of Alzheimer's disease, read *What Happens Next? A Booklet about Being Diagnosed with Alzheimer's Disease or a Related Disorder*. This booklet was written by people with a diagnosis of dementia in a support group at the Northwestern University Alzheimer's Disease Center in Chicago.

If the feelings remain strong for more than a week, however, talk with your doctor. You might be experiencing depression or anxiety.

Moving forward, consider joining an early-stage Alzheimer's disease support group. A support group can help you and your family to:

- learn about the disease
- get useful advice about living with the disease
- connect with others in similar situations
- cope with strong feelings

References

1 "Alzheimer's Disease: Unraveling the Mystery," National Institute on Aging, last updated March 20, 2014, accessed March 31, 2014, http://www.nia.nih.gov/alzheimers/publication/part-2-what-happens-brain-ad/changing-brain-ad.

2 James E. Galvin and Carl H. Sadowsky, "Practical Guidelines for the Recognition and Diagnosis of Dementia," *The Journal of the American*

Board of Family Medicine 25, no. 3 (2012), 367–82. www.jabfm.org/
content/25/3/367.long.

3   "2014 Alzheimer's Disease Facts and Figures," Alzheimer's Association,
    accessed March 31, 2014, http://www.alz.org/downloads/facts_
    figures_2014.pdf.

4   Guy M. McKhann et al, "The Diagnosis of Dementia due to Alzheimer's
    Disease: Recommendations from the National Institute on Aging-
    Alzheimer's Association Workgroups on Diagnostic Guidelines for
    Alzheimer's Disease," *Alzheimer's & Dementia* 7, no. 3 (2011), 263–9.
    doi:10.1016/j.jalz.2011.03.005.

5   "Diagnosing Alzheimer's," U.S. Department of Health and Human
    Services, accessed May 31, 2014, http://www.alzheimers.gov/
    diagnosing.html.

6   "Forgetfulness: Knowing When to Ask for Help," National Institute on
    Aging, last updated March 11, 2014, accessed March 31, 2014, http://
    www.nia.nih.gov/health/publication/forgetfulness.

7   "Alzheimer's Disease," American Academy of Neurology,
    accessed March 31, 2014, http://patients.aan.com/
    disorders/?event=view&disorder_id=844.

8   "Testing for Alzheimer's Disease: When You Need a Brain Scan—and
    When You Don't," Consumer Reports, last updated February 2013,
    accessed May 31, 2014, http://consumerhealthchoices.org/wp-content/
    uploads/2013/02/ChoosingWiselyAlzheimersSNMMI-ER.pdf.

9   "Alzheimer's Diagnostic Guidelines Updated for First Time in
    Decades," National Institute on Aging, last updated April 19, 2011,
    accessed May 31, 2014, http://www.nia.nih.gov/newsroom/2011/04/
    alzheimers-diagnostic-guidelines-updated-first-time-decades.

10 "Alzheimer's Disease Research Centers," National Institute on Aging,
    accessed May 31, 2014, http://www.nia.nih.gov/alzheimers/alzheimers-
    disease-research-centers.

11 "Just Diagnosed," Alzheimer's Association, accessed May 31, 2014,
    http://www.alz.org/i-have-alz/just-diagnosed.asp.

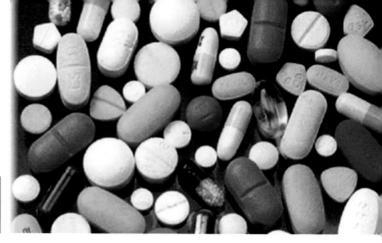

•*Alzheimer's Disease Prescription Drug Treatment*

Case Study

Violet's daughters didn't know what to expect from the medicines that were prescribed to their mother. Right after she was diagnosed with Alzheimer's disease, she began taking a medicine to help preserve her memory and thinking skills. But the drug did little to slow the progression of the disease. However, when Violet's behavior became combative (and she started kicking her daughters in the knees), an antipsychotic helped to calm her.

38. Is there a cure for Alzheimer's disease?

Today, there is no cure for Alzheimer's disease, and there is no treatment that can stop the underlying disease from progressing. However, several drugs are approved by the U.S. Food and Drug Administration (FDA) to help stabilize the disease or delay worsening of symptoms.

39. Can Alzheimer's disease be slowed or reversed?

There are no drug treatments that can slow, stop, or reverse progression of the *underlying disease* of Alzheimer's disease. However, there are four medicines that are approved by the FDA to help treat the *symptoms* of the disease (see Table 5.1). These drugs can help people with Alzheimer's to:

How long these drugs help a patient varies, from a few months to a few years.

NOTE

- Maintain thinking, memory, and speaking skills and
- Improve some behavioral and personality changes

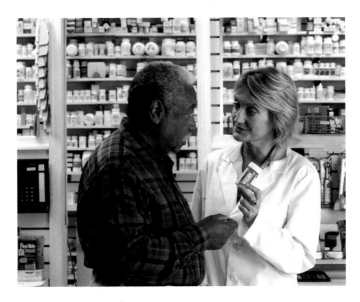

40. What are the goals of treatment?

Talk with your doctor about what you hope to achieve through treatment for Alzheimer's disease. In general, the goals of treatment are to:

- Preserve cognitive and functional ability
- Minimize behavioral disturbances
- Slow disease progression
- Ease the burden on patients and families
- Maintain quality-of-life

41. What types of health care providers treat Alzheimer's disease?

Primary care doctors are often the first ones to talk with people about memory concerns and other potential Alzheimer's disease symptoms. They are often the ones to diagnose the disease, as well.

As the U.S. population ages, more people than ever will be diagnosed with dementia. Experts think this means that family doctors will play an even bigger role in recognizing early signs and symptoms of the disease, ordering tests, diagnosing, and treating patients for Alzheimer's disease.

In addition to primary care doctors, other doctors who treat Alzheimer's disease include:

- neurologists
- internists
- geriatricians
- psychiatrists

42. What medicines are approved by the FDA to treat Alzheimer's disease?

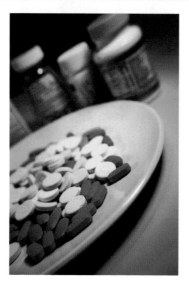

Four medicines are approved by the FDA to treat Alzheimer's disease (see Table 5.1). Each may help patients maintain thinking, memory, and speaking skills. They may also help reduce some behavioral symptoms.

These drugs may help relieve symptoms for a few months to a few years, but they do not stop the underlying disease from progressing. They regulate chemicals in the brain called neurotransmitters that transmit messages between neurons.

Table 5.1 FDA-Approved Medicines for Alzheimer's Disease

MEDICINE	USED TO TREAT MILD TO MODERATE DISEASE	USED TO TREAT MODERATE TO SEVERE DISEASE
Aricept® (donepezil)	✔	✔
Exelon® (rivastigmine)	✔	
Namenda® (memantine)		✔
Razadyne® (galantamine)	✔	

Aricept® (donepezil), Exelon® (rivastigmine), and Razadyne® (galantamine) are in a class of medicines called "cholinesterase inhibitors." Scientists aren't sure how they work to treat Alzheimer's disease, but they think that cholinesterase inhibitors help prevent the breakdown of a chemical in the brain called "acetylcholine," which may be needed for memory and thinking.

Namenda® (memantine) is in a different class of medicine, called "N-methyl D-aspartate (NMDA) antagonists." Experts think that it works by regulating a key brain chemical called "glutamate." Too much glutamate can lead to brain cell death.

Because they work in different ways, cholinesterase inhibitors can be safely used along with NMDA antagonists.

For information about specific medicines, including "Label Information," search by drug name at www.fda .gov/drugsatfda.

- Aricept® (donepezil) – www.fda.gov/Drugs and click on "Drugs @ FDA," search for Aricept, and click on drug-name links to see "Label Information"

- Exelon® (rivastigmine) - www.fda .gov/Drugs and click on "Drugs @ FDA," search for Exelon, and click on drug-name links to see "Label Information"

- Namenda® (memantine) - www .namenda.com and click on "Full Prescribing Information" to see the drug label

- Razadyne® (galantamine) - www .razadyneer.com and click on "Full Prescribing Information" to see the drug label

43. How long do Alzheimer's disease medicines work?

The medicines that are approved by the FDA to treat Alzheimer's disease may help with preserving memory, thinking, and speaking skills and certain behavioral problems for a few months to a few years.

44. What are the side effects of medicines used to treat Alzheimer's disease?

In most cases, doctors start people on low doses of Alzheimer's disease medicine and increase the dose based on how well the medicine is tolerated. This is because the higher the dose, the more likely it is that there will be unwanted side effects.

Patients should be monitored by their doctor when they start a new medicine. Any side effects or unusual symptoms should be reported to their doctor right away.

Cholinesterase inhibitors may cause mild to moderate side effects such as nausea, vomiting, and diarrhea. NMDA antagonists may cause dizziness, headache, constipation, and confusion.

Behavioral and psychiatric symptoms, which are called "neuropsychiatric" symptoms, tend to be the most difficult symptoms for people with dementia, their caregivers, and their doctors to manage. These symptoms, which can include depression, psychosis, agitation, aggression, apathy, sleep disturbance, and reduced inhibition are linked to nursing home placement, caregiver stress, hospital stays, and faster disease progression.

Often the right treatment can help reduce or stabilize behavioral and psychiatric symptoms. But prescribing the right treatment depends on figuring out what is causing the symptoms.

Sometimes symptoms can reflect an underlying infection or illness that needs to be treated; for example, the pain or discomfort of a urinary tract infection can lead to agitation. Other times, symptoms can result from side effects of medicines or from drug interactions. It's important to rule out or address these kinds of problems.

In general, non-drug strategies such as encouraging exercise and playing soothing music should be considered before treatment with medicine (see Chapter 6, Alzheimer's Disease Non-drug Treatment). This is because medicines sometimes can worsen symptoms or cause unwanted side effects. However, when non-drug strategies don't work, medicines can be an option if symptoms are so severe they outweigh the side effects or if the person might harm him- or herself or others.

When trying medicines for behavioral symptoms, keep the following in mind:

- Medicines should target specific symptoms so that their effects on those symptoms can be monitored.
- Treatment should start with a low dose of a single drug.
- Individuals should be monitored closely for side effects.
- Treatment should be for a limited amount of time because symptoms may get better over time.

Unfortunately, medicines used for behavioral and psychiatric symptoms are not likely to help with being unfriendly, taking poor care of oneself, memory problems, paying little attention to or not caring about what is going on, asking or saying the same things, not wanting care, shadowing (following or mimicking the caregiver), or wandering.

No drugs are approved by the FDA to treat behavioral and psychiatric symptoms, but several types are used (see Table 5.2). Doctors are allowed to prescribe medicine for uses not approved by the FDA for marketing.

Table 5.2 Prescription Drugs Used to Treat Behavioral and Psychiatric Symptoms of Alzheimer's Disease

ANTIDEPRESSANT MEDICINES FOR LOW MOOD AND IRRITABILITY	ANXIOLYTIC MEDICINES FOR ANXIETY, RESTLESSNESS, VERBALLY DISRUPTIVE BEHAVIOR, AND RESISTANCE	ANTIPSYCHOTIC MEDICINES FOR HALLUCINATIONS, DELUSIONS, AGGRESSION, HOSTILITY, AND UNCOOPERATIVENESS
Celexa® (citalopram)	Ativan® (lorazepam)	Abilify® (aripiprazole)
Prozac® (fluoxetine)	Serax® (oxazepam)	Zyprexa® (olanzapine)
Paxil® (paroxetine)		Seroquel® (quetiapine)
Zoloft® (sertraline)		Risperdal® (risperidone)
Desyrel® (trazodone)		Geoden® (ziprasidone)
		Haldol® (haloperidol)

SOURCE: "Behavioral Symptoms," Alzheimer's Association, accessed May 28, 2014, http://www.alz.org/professionals_and_researchers_behavioral_symptoms_pr.asp.

Drugs used to treat agitation, aggression, hallucinations, and delusions should be managed by a doctor with experience and interest in this area.

Antipsychotic drugs should be used with extreme caution. People with dementia are at risk for major side effects from these drugs, including stroke and death.

46. What prescription medicines are used to improve sleep quality?

Most doctors avoid prescribing sleep aids for people with dementia because they can cause major side effects, including incontinence, problems with balance, falls, and agitation.

Likewise, experts warn that people with dementia should not use over-the-counter sleep aids. Many contain the antihistamine Benadryl® (diphenhydramine), which further suppresses the activity of a chemical that is already reduced by Alzheimer's disease. Examples of these medicines are:

- Compoz®
- Nytol®
- Sominex®
- Unisom®
- "Nighttime" or "PM" versions of pain relievers and cold/sinus treatments

Instead, doctors may prescribe the antidepressant Desyrel® (trazodone), because it makes people sleepy in addition to helping with depression. They sometimes prescribe anti-anxiety medicines too.

47. What research is under way to improve treatment for Alzheimer's disease?

In 2012, the U.S. Federal government announced the National Plan to Address Alzheimer's Disease. This plan set goals for finding ways to prevent, treat, halt, or even reverse the disease by 2025. To meet this goal, partnerships have been forged between the National Institutes of Health, research centers at universities, and the pharmaceutical industry.

One area for which research funds have been allotted is advancing our knowledge about how genes are involved in Alzheimer's disease, including:

- identifying rare genetic variants that protect against or increase the risk of Alzheimer's disease
- exploring differences in data from different racial and ethnic groups
- examining how brain images and other biomarkers are linked with genome sequences

In addition, the National Institutes of Health, 10 biopharmaceutical companies and several nonprofit organizations have teamed up to identify and confirm promising biological targets most likely to respond to new therapies for Alzheimer's disease and other chronic diseases. The five-year initiative is called the Accelerating Medicines Partnership.

To learn more about the National Plan to Address Alzheimer's Disease, including an update for 2014, visit

http://aspe.hhs.gov/daltcp/napa/NatlPlan2014.shtml

To learn more about the Accelerating Medicines Partnership, visit

http://www.nih.gov/science/amp/alzheimers.htm.

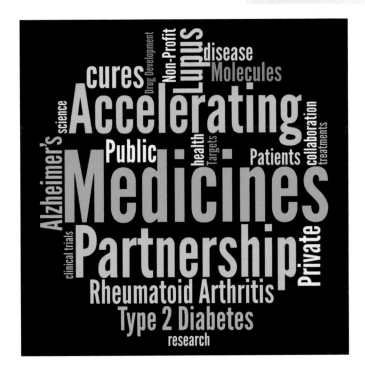

48. What is a clinical trial, and how can I take part in one?

Clinical trials are research studies that test the safety, side effects, or effectiveness of a medicine or other treatment in people. Study volunteers who want to help increase knowledge about Alzheimer's disease can take part in these studies. The results help to improve the prevention and treatment of the disease.

To learn about clinical trials:

- Talk with your doctor
- Visit NIH Clinical Research Trials and You at www.nih
  .gov/health/clinicaltrials
- Watch "Alzheimer's Disease Clinical Trials: Dr. Laurie
  Ryan" at http://www.youtube.com/watch?v=Fmjstx6JHS8

To find a clinical trial near you:

- Call the Alzheimer's Disease Education and Referral
  (ADEAR) Center at 1-800-438-4380 or visit it online at
  http://www.nia.nih.gov/alzheimers/clinical-trials
- Visit www.ClinicalTrials.gov
- Try the Alzheimer's Associations' TrialMatch®, a free
  service that matches people
  with Alzheimer's disease,
  caregivers, healthy volunteers,
  and physicians with studies. Call
  this service at 1-800-272-3900 or
  visit online at https://trialmatch
  .alz.org.

"Participating in Alzheimer's Disease Clinical Trials and Studies Fact Sheet" explains the scientific design of clinical trials and offers key facts and questions to consider if you're thinking about volunteering for clinical research.

ON THE CD

49. How can I prepare for doctor appointments?

Because the symptoms of Alzheimer's disease change over time, people with the disease should see their doctor on a regular basis so that treatment strategies can be adapted to meet their current needs.

To get the most out of doctor's visits, a family member, close friend, or caregiver should come to all visits to help ask and answer questions. In addition, follow these tips:

- Make appointments for a time at which the person with
  Alzheimer's disease can be most at ease
- Bring a list of the prescription and over-the-counter
  drugs and supplements the patient is taking, or the
  actual bottles, to help the doctor check for potential side
  effects and drug interactions
- Take time to reflect on new living routines or living
  situations, as well as changes in mood, memory, or
  abilities that have happened since the last doctor visit

- Come prepared with specific examples of things that concern you
- Ask the doctor to write down the meanings of any medical words that are hard to understand
- Before leaving, try to repeat back what the doctor said using your own words. This way the doctor can correct you if he or she was not clear enough the first time

To get ready for doctor's appointments, fill out the Alzheimer's Association's checklist, "Preparing for Your Doctor's Visit." It includes prompts about changes in mood and memory and problems with daily activities, as well as a list of helpful questions to ask the doctor.

References

1   James E. Galvin and Carl H. Sadowsky, "Practical Guidelines for the Recognition and Diagnosis of Dementia," *The Journal of the American Board of Family Medicine,* 25, no. 3 (2012), 367–82. www.jabfm.org/content/25/3/367.long.

2   "Alzheimer's Disease," American Academy of Neurology, accessed March 31, 2014, http://patients.aan.com/disorders/?event=view&disorder_id=844.

3   "Forgetfulness: Knowing When to Ask for Help," National Institute on Aging, last updated March 11, 2014, accessed November 8, 2013, http://www.nia.nih.gov/health/publication/forgetfulness.

4   "About Alzheimer's Disease: Treatment," National Institute on Aging, accessed May 28, 2014, http://www.nia.nih.gov/alzheimers/topics/treatment.

5   "Alzheimer's Disease Medications Fact Sheet," National Institute on Aging, last updated December 17, 2014, accessed August 10, 2011, http://www.nia.nih.gov/alzheimers/publication/alzheimers-disease-medications-fact-sheet.

6   Helen C. Kales, Laura N. Gitlin, Constantine G. Lyketsos, and the Detroit Expert Panel on the Assessment and Management of the Neuropsychiatric Symptoms of Dementia. "Management of Neuropsychiatric Symptoms of Dementia in Clinical Settings: Recommendations from a Multidisciplinary Expert Panel." *Journal of the American Geriatrics Society* 62, no. 4 (2014): 762–69. http://doi.wiley.com/10.1111/jgs.12730.

7   "Behavioral Symptoms," Alzheimer's Association, accessed May 28, 2014, http://www.alz.org/professionals_and_researchers_behavioral_symptoms_pr.asp.

8   Jason Karlawish, "How Are We Going to Live with Alzheimer's Disease?" *Health Affairs* 33, no. 4 (2014), 541–6, accessed May 31, 2014, http://content.healthaffairs.org/content/33/4/541.full.

9   "NIH Funds Next Step of Cutting-Edge Research into Alzheimer's Disease Genome," National Institutes of Health, last updated July 7, 2014, accessed July 7, 2014, http://www.nih.gov/news/health/jul2014/nia-07.htm.

10   "Understanding Memory Loss: What to Do When You Have Trouble Remembering," National Institute on Aging, last updated October 6, 2014, accessed May 29, 2014, http://www.nia.nih.gov/alzheimers/publication/understanding-memory-loss/help-serious-memory-problems.

11   "Medical Management & Patient Care," Alzheimer's Association, accessed May 28, 2014, http://www.alz.org/health-care-professionals/medical-management-patient-care.asp.

12   "Doctor's Visits," Alzheimer's Society of Canada, last updated December 2, 2013, accessed July 25, 2014, http://www.alzheimer.ca/en/About-dementia/Diagnosis/Getting-a-diagnosis/Doctor-s-visits.

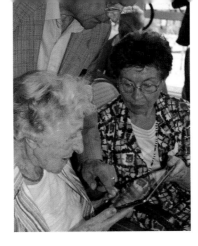

Alzheimer's Disease Nondrug Treatment •

Case Study

When Violet was in the moderate stages of Alzheimer's disease, she still was able to enjoy many activities. One favorite was going for walks in the neighborhood with her daughters. During their walks together, Violet would become more engaged and talkative—a sign that she was enjoying herself. She also loved doing crossword puzzles. Many people with Alzheimer's disease who once enjoyed puzzles still do when in the early to moderate stages of the disease. Her daughters would bring her stacks of crossword puzzle books from the discount store. She also liked to draw and write, which were activities that were set up in the assisted living home. Her daughters might not have known it at the time—they were simply trying to find pleasurable moments for their mom—but exercise and stimulation enhance cognitive and social functioning.

50. What nondrug interventions can help with behavioral and psychiatric symptoms?

There are many nondrug interventions that can help improve behavioral and psychiatric symptoms. The goals of these treatments are prevention, symptom relief, and reduction of caregiver stress. In fact, experts recommend that nondrug treatments be tried first, before drug-based interventions.

In most cases, managing behavioral and psychiatric symptoms includes:

- identifying the behavior
- understanding its cause
- adapting the caregiving environment to address the situation

Often, the right intervention can help reduce or stabilize behavioral and psychiatric symptoms. But figuring out what is causing them is key to proper treatment. Sometimes symptoms can reflect an underlying infection or illness that needs to be treated; for example, the pain or discomfort of a urinary tract infection can lead to agitation. Other times, symptoms can result from side effects of medicines or drug interactions. It's important to address or rule out these kinds of problems.

Some people call nondrug interventions "behavioral and environmental interventions."

To help identify what might be causing behavioral and psychiatric symptoms, your doctor may:

- ask you to bring a list of prescription and over-the-counter drugs and supplements or the actual bottles
- check for common health problems, such as urinary tract infection, constipation, dehydration, and pain
- take blood samples to check factors such as blood sugar level and electrolytes
- ask about a prior mental health history, such as anxiety or depression
- check for sensory impairments, like poor hearing or vision

In many cases, however, it is a change in the person's environment that triggers the symptoms (see Table 6.1). Bathing and changing clothes can trigger symptoms, as well.

Table 6.1 Environmental Changes That Might Trigger Symptoms

Change of caregiver
Change in living arrangements
Travel
Hospitalization
Presence of houseguests

SOURCE: "Behavioral Symptoms," Alzheimer's Association, accessed May 31, 2014, http://www.alz.org/professionals_and_researchers_behavioral_symptoms_pr.asp.

There are many general nondrug strategies to help reduce symptoms brought about by these types of changes, including the following:

- Redirect the person's attention, rather than argue or disagree
- Simplify the environment (e.g., remove clutter, reduce noise)
- Simplify tasks and routines
- Allow rest time between stimulating events
- Use labels to cue or remind the person (e.g., arrows pointing to bathroom)
- Use lighting to reduce confusion and restlessness at night

A doctor can advise you about what specific behavioral and psychiatric strategies might help with the symptoms that are most troublesome (see Table 6.2).

Table 6.2 Nondrug Strategies to Improve Specific Behavioral and Psychiatric Symptoms

SYMPTOMS	STRATEGIES
Apathy	Provide stimulation Encourage activities Provide simple tasks
Nighttime wakefulness	Encourage daily activity and exercise Promote good sleep hygiene (e.g., going to bed at the same time every night and making the bedroom quiet, dark, and at a comfortable temperature) Provide daytime stimulation Provide less stimulation in the evening Eliminate caffeine Provide a quiet bedtime routine (e.g., calming activities and music) Use a nightlight Limit daytime napping
Irritability/ Agitation	Redirect attention (e.g., change the subject or activity) Break down tasks into simple steps See question 51 for more ideas
Wandering	Identify when wandering is most likely to occur and plan activities for those times Use visual cues (e.g., arrows pointing to the bathroom or a stop sign on the front door) Encourage exercise Provide safe places to wander

(continued)

Table 6.2 Continued

SYMPTOMS	STRATEGIES
Mood disorders	Encourage exercise
Psychotic symptoms	Remove mirrors Reassure Distract instead of confront
Eating/Appetite Problems	Offer simple finger foods Remove distractions from dining area Play soothing music
Aggression	Identify and modify underlying cause of aggression Avoid confronting or being physical Use self-protection strategies (back away, distract, leave patient alone if patient is safe, and seek help) Remove dangerous items Create a calm, soothing environment (e.g., remove clutter and lessen noise)

SOURCE: Helen C. Kales, Laura N. Gitlin, Constantine G. Lyketsos, and the Detroit Expert Panel on the Assessment and Management of the Neuropsychiatric Symptoms of Dementia. "Management of Neuropsychiatric Symptoms of Dementia in Clinical Settings: Recommendations from a Multidisciplinary Expert Panel," *Journal of the American Geriatrics Society* 62, no. 4 (2014): 762–9. http://doi.wiley.com/10.1111/jgs.12730.

SOURCE: Freddi Segal-Gidan et al. "Alzheimer's Disease Management Guideline: Update 2008." Alzheimer's & Dementia, 7, no. 3 (May 2011): e51–e59. http://www.ncbi.nlm.nih.gov/pubmed/21546322.

If these types of strategies don't work, medicine might be an option if symptoms are severe or if the person might harm him- or herself or others (see Chapter 5, Alzheimer's Disease Prescription Drug Treatment). Nonetheless, medicine should be used along with nondrug approaches.

51. What nondrug interventions can help with agitation?

Research suggests that music can reduce agitation during baths.

Agitation is common among people with Alzheimer's disease but many caregiver strategies can help prevent and defuse it. The Alzheimer's Association recommends these dos and don'ts, and what you might say to lessen agitation (see Table 6.3).

There are also a number of ways to help prevent agitation in the first place, including those listed in Table 6.4.

Table 6.3 Strategies to Use During an Episode of Agitation

DO	DON'T	SAY
• Back off and ask permission • Use calm, positive statements • Reassure • Slow down • Add light • Offer guided choices between two options • Focus on pleasant events • Offer simple exercise options • Limit stimulation	• Raise your voice • Take offense • Corner, crowd, or restrain • Rush • Criticize or shame • Ignore • Force or demand • Confront or argue • Reason • Condescend • Explain or teach • Show alarm • Make sudden movements out of the person's view	• May I help you? • Do you have time to help me? • You're safe here. • Everything is under control. • I apologize. • I'm sorry that you are upset. • I know it's hard. • I will stay until you feel better.

Source: "Behavioral Symptoms," Alzheimer's Association, accessed May 31, 2014, http://www.alz.org/professionals_and_researchers_behavioral_symptoms_pr.asp.

Table 6.4 Strategies to Prevent Agitation

CREATE A CALM ENVIRONMENT	AVOID ENVIRONMENTAL TRIGGERS	MONITOR PERSONAL COMFORT
• Remove stressors, triggers, or danger • Move person to a safer or quieter place • Change expectations	• Noise • Glare • Unsecure space • Too much background distraction, including television	Ask about or check for signs of • Pain • Hunger • Thirst • Constipation • Full bladder • Fatigue • Infections • Skin irritation

(continued)

Table 6.4 Continued

CREATE A CALM ENVIRONMENT	AVOID ENVIRONMENTAL TRIGGERS	MONITOR PERSONAL COMFORT
• Offer security object, rest, or privacy • Limit caffeine use • Provide opportunity for exercise • Develop soothing rituals • Use gentle reminders		Ensure a comfortable temperature Be sensitive to • Fears • Misperceived threats • Frustration with attempts to express what is wanted

SOURCE: "Behavioral Symptoms," Alzheimer's Association, accessed May 31, 2014, http://www.alz.org/professionals_and_researchers_behavioral_symptoms_pr.asp.

52. Are there ways to help boost memory?

Large calendars, a list of daily plans, notes about simple safety measures, and simple directions for using common household items are useful memory aids.

There are a variety of ways to help people with early Alzheimer's disease maintain their memory and mental skills, including these:

- Plan ahead. Make to-do lists and use memory aids like notes and calendars.
- Encourage interests or hobbies; keep up with activities that engages the mind and body.
- Encourage physically activity and exercise. Walking is a good option.
- Limit alcohol intake.
- Relieve stress, anxiety, or depression with activities like exercise and hobbies. If these feeling persist, talk with the patient's doctor.

53. Is occupational therapy helpful?

Occupational therapy helps people of all ages do the daily tasks they need and want to do. For people with Alzheimer's disease, the goals are to maximize quality of life and to balance safety with independence.

In most cases, occupational services include:

- an evaluation, during which the person and his or her caregivers determine the goals of therapy
- a personalized intervention to improve the person's ability to perform everyday activities and achieve his or her goals
- follow-up appointments to check that the goals are being met and to make any necessary changes to the interventions

Occupational therapy can be helpful throughout the course of Alzheimer's disease: from early on, when everyday activities become difficult or dangerous, to later stages of the disease, to help assist with self-care and difficult behaviors.

Occupational therapists analyze tasks involved in everyday activities and adapt them to make them achievable by:

- reducing the number of steps required
- simplifying procedures
- setting up the task so it is ready to begin
- completing portions of the task beforehand (e.g., starting the task or doing the more difficult parts)
- controlling the environment (e.g., clearing a space for the task or providing task lighting)

They also will learn about the main living space (often called the "physical environment") in which the person with Alzheimer's disease lives so that supports can be provided to increase safety and functioning and to prevent slips and falls, burns, poisonings, cuts, electrocution, and drowning. Examples of supports to prevent slips and falls include creating workspaces where the person can sit during activities and adding bathroom grab bars or railings.

Because Alzheimer's disease is a progressive condition, the focus of occupational therapy is not on new learning for the patient but on education for the caregiver, making changes to the environment, and compensatory strategies.

ON THE WEB

To learn about the various occupational therapy interventions that are recommended for people with Alzheimer's disease, read "Occupational Therapy Practice Guidelines for Adults with Alzheimer's Disease and Related Disorders" from the American Occupational Therapy Association at

http://www.guideline.gov

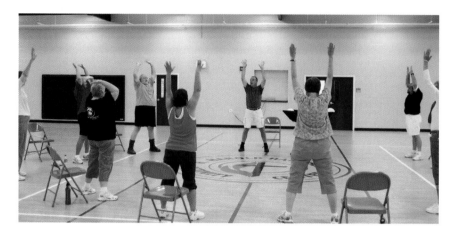

Research has shown that exercise can help to:

- improve or maintain strength and fitness
- prevent or treat many health problems, including arthritis, heart disease, diabetes, and high blood pressure
- lessen balance problems and trouble walking

For inspiration, exercise charts, and comprehensive information on how to get started, reduce risks, and reward progress, read "Exercise & Physical Activity: Your Everyday Guide from the National Institute on Aging."

ON THE CD

For ideas about how to boost physical activity levels in people with Alzheimer's disease, read "Activity and Exercise RX for Persons with Alzheimer's" from the National Center on Health, Physical Activity and Disability at

ON THE WEB

http://www.nchpad.org/116/901/Alzheimer~s~Disease.

It can also help with feelings of depression or anxiety and can lift your mood. In fact, there are few downsides to physical activity if it is done within your physical abilities.

But it is also thought to aid cognitive function and to potentially improve or delay the symptoms of Alzheimer's disease. In fact, a 2013 review of 16 clinical studies, conducted by the Cochrane Collaboration, found promising evidence that exercise programs can improve cognitive functioning and the ability to perform daily activities in people with dementia.

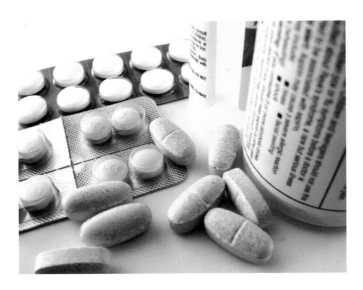

Many complementary and alternative therapies have been studied to see if they can help prevent or slow the effect of Alzheimer's disease.

Some dietary supplements claim to enhance memory or improve brain function. But so far, no strong evidence has emerged that shows that any dietary supplements are effective for Alzheimer's disease. This includes ginkgo biloba, omega-3 fatty acids/fish oil, vitamins B and E, Asian ginseng, grape seed extract, and curcumin (a chemical found in turmeric). However, more research is being done on some of these supplements.

Because supplements can interact with medicines and can have serious side effects, be sure to talk with your doctor before taking any.

To learn about the results of research on specific supplements, visit the National Center for Complementary and Integrative Medicine at

http://nccih.nih.gov/health/providers/digest/alzheimers-science

Early studies of some mind and body practices suggest that they might reduce some Alzheimer's disease symptoms. For example, several studies have shown that music therapy improves agitation, depression, and quality of life. Mental imagery is another mind and body practice that has shown promise in preliminary studies.

56. What is cognitive training, and does it work?

Cognitive training is a type of nondrug intervention that is used in early-stage dementia to help make the most of memory and cognitive function. It involves guided practice on a set of tasks that exercise memory, attention, or problem-solving. The guiding assumption is that practice can improve or maintain function.

Cognitive training tasks can be paper-based, done on the computer, or simulate activities of daily living. It can be done one-on-one or in groups, and sessions typically last up to an hour each, at least once per week.

Some experts believe that cognitive training may help slow the effects of Alzheimer's disease, especially among early-onset patients, because the brain has the ability to reorganize and repair itself to some degree, even after being damaged.

Cognitive training is also known as cognitive retraining, cognitive remediation, or brain training.

Although some studies have found that cognitive training can improve cognitive function among people with Alzheimer's disease, a 2013 review of 11 studies from the Cochrane Collaboration found no support for its effectiveness in improving cognitive function.

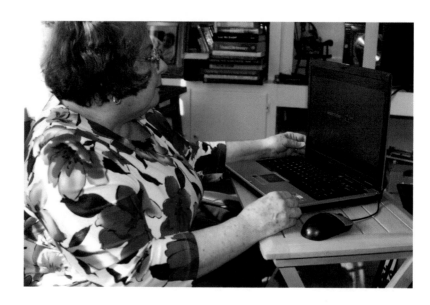

1   Helen C. Kales, Laura N. Gitlin, Constantine G. Lyketsos, and the Detroit Expert Panel on the Assessment and Management of the Neuropsychiatric Symptoms of Dementia. "Management of Neuropsychiatric Symptoms of Dementia in Clinical Settings: Recommendations from a Multidisciplinary Expert Panel," *Journal of the American Geriatrics Society* 62, no. 4 (2014): 762–9. http://doi.wiley.com/10.1111/jgs.12730.

2   "Behavioral Symptoms," Alzheimer's Association, accessed May 31, 2014, http://www.alz.org/professionals_and_researchers_behavioral_symptoms_pr.asp.

3   Anton P. Porsteinsson et al., "Effect of Citalopram on Agitation in Alzheimer Disease: The CitAD Randomized Clinical Trial," *JAMA* 311, no. 7 (2014): 682–9. http://jama.jamanetwork.com/article.aspx?articleid=1829989.

4   Constantine G. Lyketsos et al., "Neuropsychiatric Symptoms in Alzheimer's Disease." *Alzheimer's & Dementia: The Journal of the Alzheimer's Association* 7, no. 5 (2011), 532–9. www.alzheimersanddementia.com/article/S1552-5260(11)02575-1/abstract.

5   "Forgetfulness: Knowing When to Ask for Help," National Institute on Aging, last updated March 11, 2014, accessed March 31, 2014, http://www.nia.nih.gov/health/publication/forgetfulness.

6   "Occupational Therapy Practice Guidelines for Adults with Alzheimer's Disease and Related Disorders," National Guideline Clearinghouse, accessed June 2, 2014, http://www.guideline.gov/content.aspx?id=16321&search=alzheimer%27s+disease.

7   "About Occupational Therapy," American Occupational Therapy Association, accessed July 13, 2014, http://www.aota.org/about-occupational-therapy.aspx.

8   "Exercise & Physical Activity: Your Everyday Guide from the National Institute on Aging," National Institute on Aging, accessed July 18, 2011. http://www.nia.nih.gov/health/publication/exercise-physical-activity/introduction.

9   Keith A. Wollen, "Pharmaceutical, Nutritional, Botanical, and Stimulatory Therapies, with a Discussion of Treatment Strategies from the Perspective of Patients and Practitioners." *Alternative Medicine Review: A Journal of Clinical Therapeutics,* 15, no. 3 (2010): 223–44. http://www.altmedrev.com.ezproxy.library.tufts.edu/publications/15/3/223.pdf.

10 Dorothy Forbes et al. "Exercise Programs for People with Dementia," in *Cochrane Database of Systematic Reviews* (John Wiley & Sons, Ltd, 1996) . http://onlinelibrary.wiley.com/doi/10.1002/14651858.CD006489.pub3/abstract.

11   "Alzheimer's Disease at a Glance," National Center for Complementary and Alternative Medicine, accessed July 11, 2014, http://nccam.nih.gov/health/alzheimer/ataglance.

12   "5 Things To Know About Complementary Health Practices for Cognitive Function, Dementia, and Alzheimer's Disease," National Center for Complementary and Alternative Medicine, accessed July 11, 2014, http://nccam.nih.gov/health/tips/alzheimers.

13   Alex Bahar-Fuchs, Linda Clare, and Bob Woods, "Cognitive training and cognitive rehabilitation for mild to moderate Alzheimer's disease and vascular dementia (review)". *The Cochrane Database of Systematic Reviews* 6 (June 5, 2013). http://onlinelibrary.wiley.com/doi/10.1002/14651858.CD003260.pub2/abstract;jsessionid=33E4757E38E12DEB3FCF7757CB10A85C.f03t04. .

14   Fang Yu et al. "Cognitive training for early-stage Alzheimer's disease and dementia." *Journal of Gerontological Nursing,* 35, no. 3 (2009), 23–9.

15   Freddi Segal-Gidan et al., "Alzheimer's Disease Management Guideline: Update 2008." Alzheimer's & Dementia, 7, no. 3 (May 2011): e51–e59. http://www.ncbi.nlm.nih.gov/pubmed/21546322.

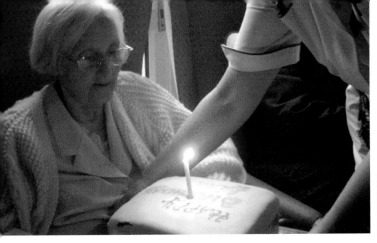

Living with Alzheimer's Disease •————

Making sure that their mother was safe was a priority for Violet's daughters. They put medicine higher than she could reach so she couldn't accidentally take too much, added extra locks on the doors so she couldn't wander, and took her car keys away after she ended up across town on a trip to a nearby store. They also took the knobs off the stove and unplugged the oven, which meant that her daughters would need to supply cooked meals for her from then on.

57. Is eating a healthy diet important in Alzheimer's disease?

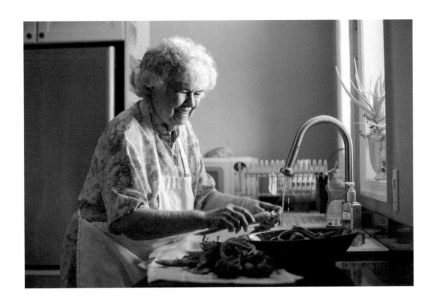

To learn more about eating a healthy diet, including a video on nutrient-dense foods, visit

ON THE WEB

http://nihseniorhealth.gov/ eatingwellasyougetolder and select "Choose Nutrient-dense Foods."

Experts think that a heart-healthy diet may protect the brain from Alzheimer's disease. But eating well has not been linked with improvement of the symptoms of the disease. Nonetheless, a healthy diet has many benefits. It may reduce the risk of heart disease, stroke, diabetes, bone loss, some cancers, and anemia.

To eat a healthy diet, choose:

- fruits and vegetables
- grains, especially whole grains
- low-fat or fat-free dairy products
- seafood, lean poultry and meats, beans, eggs, and unsalted nuts

But limit your intake of:

- solid fats
- cholesterol
- salt
- added sugar

58. How can we make mealtimes easier?

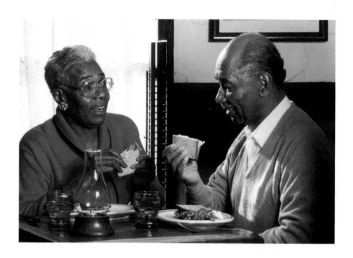

As Alzheimer's disease progresses, mealtimes can become challenging for people with the disease and for their caregivers. It's important to make the most of mealtimes, however, because staying nourished and hydrated is important for both health and well-being. What's more, mealtimes help orient people to the time of day.

Eating-related challenges can arise from many factors, including forgetting to eat, not wanting to sit down for meals, not being able to tell the plate from the food, decreased appetite caused by medicines, and difficulty holding utensils.

Mealtimes can be modified in many ways to make them a successful experience for individuals and their caregivers (see Table 7.1)

 NOTE

Many people with Alzheimer's disease lose weight, and good nutrition may not be enough to prevent this.

Table 7.1 Tips for Successful Mealtimes

Encourage individuals to participate in mealtime tasks • Help prepare food • Set the table • Pull out chairs • Put dishes away
Provide mealtime cues • Eat meals together • Set the table • Use aromas to trigger appetite • Ask questions about the meal (e.g., food preferences)
To promote independence offer finger foods, which don't require utensils and are easier to eat, such as: • Small sandwiches • Cheese • Hard-boiled eggs • Cut fresh fruits and vegetables
Maintain familiar routines and adapt them as needed • Serve meals at the same times as always • Follow personal, cultural, and religious food preferences
Minimize distractions • Turn off the television and radio • Clear the table of non-food items
Offer appealing foods with familiar flavors, varied textures, and different colors

Watch a video with tips on eating called "Simplifying Mealtimes" at

http://nihseniorhealth.gov/videolist .html#caringforsomeonewithalzheimers

ON THE WEB

Keep people with dementia up to date about what time of day it is, where they live, and what is happening at home and in the world.

NOTE

59. What strategies help with memory problems?

Simple strategies can help people with memory problems keep up their everyday routines and live as normal a life as possible. In addition to telling someone what time it is, where he or she lives, and when to take his or her medicine, you can create written reminders for them. Most people with Alzheimer's disease can still read.

Memory aids can help, such as:

- big calendars to highlight important dates and events
- lists of the plans for each day
- notes about safety in the home
- written directions for using common household items

For more tips on how to handle day-to-day challenges, read "Tips for Daily Life" from the Alzheimer's Association.

ON THE CD

You can also use labeling and visual cues, such as arrows that point the way to the bathroom.

60. How do I keep a safe home for someone with Alzheimer's disease?

Having a safe home is important for all people, but those with Alzheimer's disease need to have extra precautions in place to make sure that they cannot leave home easily, don't have access to dangerous objects like knives or guns, and can move from one room to the next safely.

It is easier and more effective to modify the living environment than to try to change the behavior. And a safe home can put the person with Alzheimer's and his or her caregiver at ease.

Strategies include:

- displaying emergency numbers and your home address near all telephones
- putting safety locks on doors and gates

- removing guns and sharp knives
- installing extra smoke alarms
- controlling access to the stove
- installing grab bars
- providing adequate lighting
- removing clutter

For information about home safety, including a comprehensive, room-by-room checklist, read "Home Safety for People with Alzheimer's Disease at

http://www.nia.nih.gov/alzheimers/publication.

If the person with Alzheimer's disease tends to wander, notify your neighbors and police about the person's condition and be sure he or she wears an identification bracelet or pendant. MedicAlert® + Alzheimer's Association Safe Return® is a 24-hour nationwide emergency response system for people with

To learn more about this program, visit

http://www.alz.org/care/dementia-medic-alert-safe-return.asp.

Alzheimer's disease. If someone with Alzheimer's disease wanders, caregivers can call an emergency response line to activate local Alzheimer's Association chapters and law enforcement agencies. In addition, if a citizen or emergency worker finds the person, he or she can call the toll-free number on the person's MedicAlert + Safe Return ID jewelry.

61. What do I need to know about dental care for someone with Alzheimer's disease?

Oral health is often overlooked in the elderly and maybe even more so among those with dementia, so dental problems often go undetected. Oral health declines along with the progression of Alzheimer's disease, and dental problems and pain can lead to not wanting to eat, not wearing dentures, and aggression.

Factors that may contribute to dental problems in people with Alzheimer's disease include:

- taking medicines that cause dry mouth
- swallowing and dietary problems
- poor oral hygiene
- difficulty wearing dentures
- inability to carry out tasks needed to take care of themselves, such as oral hygiene procedures

Experts suggest that dental treatment be provided early in the course of Alzheimer's disease, with the goal of producing stable oral health. This will help keep oral health from getting worse as

Alzheimer's disease progresses and dental treatment becomes more difficult to provide.

62. What strategies help with sleep problems?

Problems with sleep are very common among people with Alzheimer's disease because the disease affects the sleep/wake cycle. Early in the disease, people may sleep more than usual or wake up disoriented. But later in the disease, they may sleep during the day and wake up often at night.

Learn how to create an ideal sleep environment from the National Sleep Foundation at

ON THE WEB

http://sleepfoundation.org/bedroom/.

Studies have found that light therapy, melatonin, and a type of therapy called "cognitive behavioral therapy" (CBT) for insomnia may help people with Alzheimer's disease sleep better at night.

Tips to help with sleep problems include the following:

- Keep a schedule as much as possible, getting the person up in the morning and going to sleep at night at the same time each day. Keeping the same meal schedule helps keep routines on track, too.
- Expose the person to bright light as often as possible during the day by going outside, especially in the morning.
- Keep the bedroom dark and quiet at night, using only a nightlight if needed.
- Encourage exercise, such as short walks or throwing a beach ball.
- Limit napping during the day to less than one hour.
- Limit caffeine, including products like coffee, tea, chocolate, and soda.

63. When is it time for someone with Alzheimer's disease to stop driving?

Studies suggest that older drivers with dementia are more likely to have accidents than other drivers and that even drivers with mild dementia are more likely to make errors and have "close calls."

Many of the symptoms of Alzheimer's disease affect driving ability and can lead to dangerous driving situations, such as:

- driving too slowly
- stopping for no reason
- not observing traffic signs or signals
- getting lost
- using poor judgment in dangerous situations
- driving while drowsy

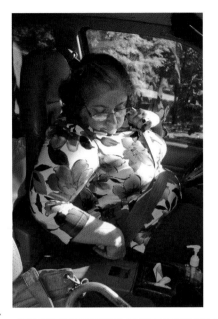

Nonetheless, a diagnosis of mild or early-stage Alzheimer's disease does not necessarily mean that a person should stop driving right away. However, because driving ability will eventually become impaired in people with Alzheimer's disease, they should have regular on-road testing of their driving skills.

To determine whether it is time for a relative with Alzheimer's disease to stop driving, families can request a formal driving evaluation by a trained professional. The evaluation should include an on-road driving component, which is thought to be the best way to evaluate driving ability.

Giving up driving is hard for many people, who perceive it as a threat to their independence. In some cases it may be easier for this information to be delivered by a physician, whose opinions may be taken more seriously than the caregiver's. Using a prescription pad, doctors can "prescribe" that patients no longer drive if they pose a risk to themselves or others on the road.

For more information about planning to stop driving, visit the Alzheimer's Association's Dementia and Driving Resource Center at

http://www.alz.org/care/alzheimers-dementia-and-driving.asp.

64. How can we make bathing easier?

Bathing can be a difficult task for someone with Alzheimer's disease. Even so, many people don't want help because they consider it a private activity. Some people may also be fearful of bathing or angry about needing help.

To help make bath time easier, follow these tips:

- Check the water temperature before beginning bathing.
- Use a hand-held showerhead, a rubber bath mat, and safety bars.
- Have all your supplies ready beforehand, such as soap, shampoo, washcloth, and towels.

A full shower or bath two or three times per week is sufficient. In between, sponge baths to clean the face, hands, feet, underarms, and genitals is all the person needs.

- Tell the person what you are going to do, step by step.
- Give the person a washcloth to hold; he or she will be less likely to hit you.
- Place a towel over the person's shoulders or lap so he or she feels less exposed.

References

1 "Taking Care of Yourself," Alzheimer's Association, accessed July 30, 2014, http://www.alz.org/i-have-alz/taking-care-of-yourself.asp.

2 "Eating Well As You Get Older," NIHSeniorHealth, last updated May 2012, accessed July 30, 2014, http://nihseniorhealth.gov/eatingwellasyougetolder/choosenutrientdensefoods/01.html.

3 "Encouraging Eating: Advice for At-Home Dementia Caregivers," National Institute on Aging, last updated June 26, 2013, accessed July 13, 2011, http://www.nia.nih.gov/alzheimers/features/encouraging-eating-advice-home-dementia-caregivers.

4 "Understanding Memory Loss," National Institute on Aging, last updated October 6, 2014, accessed March 31, 2014, http://www.nia.nih.gov/alzheimers/publication/understanding-memory-loss/help-serious-memory-problems.

5 Helen C. Kales, Laura N. Gitlin, Constantine G. Lyketsos, and the Detroit Expert Panel on the Assessment and Management of the Neuropsychiatric Symptoms of Dementia. "Management of Neuropsychiatric Symptoms of Dementia in Clinical Settings: Recommendations from a Multidisciplinary Expert Panel." *Journal of the American Geriatrics Society* 62, no. 4 (2014), 762–9. doi:10.1111/jgs.12730.

6 "Behavioral Symptoms," Alzheimer's Association, accessed May 31, 2014, http://www.alz.org/professionals_and_researchers_behavioral_symptoms_pr.asp.

7 Jane Chalmers and Alan Pearson, "Oral Hygiene Care for Residents with Dementia: A Literature Review," *Journal of Advanced Nursing* 52, no. 4 (2005): 410–9.

8   Mancini, M. et al, "Oral Health in Alzheimers Disease: A Review." *Current Alzheimer Research* 7, no. 4 (2010), 368–73. http://www.eurekaselect.com/86102/article.

9   "Alzheimer's Disease and Sleep," National Sleep Foundation, accessed July 30, 2014 http://sleepfoundation.org/sleep-disorders-problems/alzheimers-disease-and-sleep.

10 "Sleep and Alzheimer's Disease," National Sleep Foundation, accessed July 30, 2014 http://sleepfoundation.org/ask-the-expert/sleep-and-alzheimers-disease/page/0%2C1/.

11 Constantine G. Lyketsos et al., "Neuropsychiatric Symptoms in Alzheimer's Disease." *Alzheimer's & Dementia: The Journal of the Alzheimer's Association* 7, no. :5 (2011), 532–9. www.alzheimersanddementia.com/article/S1552-5260(11)02575-1/abstract.

12 "Driving and Dementia: Health Professionals Can Play Important Role," National Institute on Aging, last updated December 8, 2011, accessed July 19, 2011, http://www.nia.nih.gov/alzheimers/features/driving-and-dementia-health-professionals-can-play-important-role.

13 "Occupational Therapy Practice Guidelines for Adults with Alzheimer's Disease and Related Disorders," National Guideline Clearinghouse, last updated November 19, 2010, accessed June 2, 2014, http://www.guideline.gov/content.aspx?id=16321&search=alzheimer%27s+disease.

14 "Alzheimer's Caregiving Tips--Bathing," National Institute on Aging, last updated October 2012, accessed July 31, 2014, http://www.nia.nih.gov/sites/default/files/caregivingtips_bathing_final_12oct09_0.pdf.

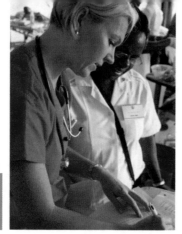

•*Being a Caregiver*

Case Study

Violet's husband did his best to care for her, but his health problems made it difficult. Because of this, Violet's daughters became her main caregivers. For them, what it means to be a caregiver has changed over the course of their mother's illness. While they still manage her financial and legal affairs, her day-to-day care—including feeding her, bathing her, and helping her use the toilet—is now provided by the professionals at the assisted living facility where she resides. With Violet in the late stage of Alzheimer's disease and unable to get out of bed, her daughters now focus on trying to connect with her. They talk to her, hold her hand, and cuddle her face. She may not recognize them, but they try to bring her joy by showing her pictures of flowers from her native Jamaica and videos of Caribbean music on their smartphones. In these moments, her eyes light up and focus, and with the music playing, she sways ever so slightly, dancing.

65. What is a caregiver?

Caregivers are the people who provide most of the care for people with illnesses. About 15 million people care for a loved one with Alzheimer's disease in the United States. Among people with Alzheimer's disease who reside at home, the main caregivers are usually their spouses and other relatives, along with key members of their health care teams.

In Alzheimer's disease, caregivers do many things, including:

- Assisting in activities of daily living, including eating, bathing, grooming, and dressing
- Providing activities and stimulation

- Managing medicines and medical, dental, and psychiatric care
- Managing legal and financial matters
- Keeping a safe living space
- Planning for the future

In addition to the main caregivers, other people can help with daily or weekly tasks, including:

- Formal (paid) help
- Additional family members
- Friends
- Neighbors

Caregiving is often influenced by cultural factors, and the experience of caregiving and its desired outcomes varies for different ethnic groups. For more information about this read "Cultural Diversity and Caregiving" at http://www.apa.org/pi/about/publications/caregivers/faq/.

66. What is it like to be a caregiver?

Caring for a person with Alzheimer's disease is challenging, physically and emotionally. Although the caregiving experience is different for everyone, for most people it is the behavioral and psychiatric symptoms of Alzheimer's disease that present the most difficulties. These symptoms include depression, psychosis (such as having delusions and seeing or hearing things), agitation, aggression, apathy, sleep problems, and the loss of inhibition/restraint. Caregivers of people with these symptoms are more likely to feel distressed and depressed than those who aren't dealing with these symptoms.

Some caregivers feel like the person with Alzheimer's disease is acting out on purpose. But almost all people with Alzheimer's disease develop these symptoms at some point, and delusions, hallucinations, and aggression become common as the disease progresses.

Other factors that make caregiving challenging include the following:

- People with Alzheimer's disease might not recognize the extent of their impairment, especially in the middle to later stages of the disease.
- People with Alzheimer's disease might get angry with their caregivers, hurt their feelings, or forget who they are.

- The symptoms of Alzheimer's disease change over time.
- People with Alzheimer's disease eventually need care around the clock.
- Many difficult and complex decisions need to be made about short-term and long-term care for people with Alzheimer's disease.
- It may be difficult to find time to care for yourself.

The caregiver's role changes over time. As the disease progresses, the need for assistance and monitoring increases. For example, a caregiver may assist with parts of an activity at first, assist with the full task later, and have the person with Alzheimer's disease observe the task passively when he or she can no longer physically participate.

Although there are many challenges, there are also many resources. Caregivers can find emotional support, practical tips, and other resources online and in person (see Question 70, What kinds of resources exist for caregivers?). Learning about Alzheimer's disease and its stages can also help you understand and cope with the illness.

67. How does being a caregiver affect my health?

"Caregiver burden" refers to the extent that a caregiver's emotional, physical, social, and financial health are affected by caring for someone.

DEFINITION

Studies have shown that caregivers of people with Alzheimer's disease have lower health-related quality of life, higher rates of depression, and more stress and anxiety than people in the general population. Further, caregivers of people with Alzheimer's disease who have more severe behavioral and psychiatric symptoms are more likely to experience depression and greater caregiver burden than caregivers of those without such symptoms.

68. How can I protect my health?

It is critical for caregivers to take care of themselves, physically and mentally. Staying healthy will help them cope with the demands of caregiving and help them to be better caregivers. It's not easy for people to find the time to take care of their needs, so they might need to ask family members and friends to help out.

Take care of yourself by following these tips:

- Ask for help when you need it.
- Eat a healthy diet and exercise regularly.
- Join a caregiver's support group.
- Take breaks every day.
- See your doctor regularly.
- Take a caregiver education class.
- See a mental health professional for help dealing with stress and strong feelings.

69. How can I cope with difficult behavior?

Many caregivers struggle with the difficult behavior (such as repeating questions, wandering, and irritability) of the person they are caring for. Every person with Alzheimer's disease is different, and you may have to try several strategies before you find ones that work for your situation.

In general, try not to take the behavior personally, remember that the behavior is not intentional but a product of the illness, and remain calm. Also, consider that pain might be an issue. Here are some more tips:

Keep extras of items that the person is attached to or always looking for. That way one is always available.

- Let the person express him or herself and acknowledge his or her opinions.
- Respond to the emotion; the person might need reassurance.
- Keep responses simple and avoid lengthy explanations or reasons.
- Redirect the person to another activity. For example, you might ask for help with a chore.

The National Institute on Aging has over 30 tip sheets on difficult behaviors, everyday care, communication, relationships, safety, caregiver health, legal and financial issues, and end-of-life care. You'll find tips on topics from managing rummaging and hiding things to coping with the holidays. Most are available as PDFs, but many are also available to download as electronic books at

http://www.nia.nih.gov/alzheimers/topics/caregiving.

See Chapter 6, Alzheimer's Disease Non-drug Treatment for more information on how to handle specific kinds of behaviors.

Many resources exist for caregivers to help ease the burden of caregiving, which can be stressful, frightening, and overwhelming at times.

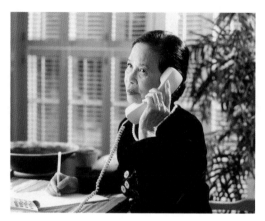

Support Groups

Support groups are a good way to stay connected to the community and seek guidance and support as a caregiver. It can be reassuring to know that you are not alone in dealing with the everyday stresses and challenges of being a caregiver. It can also be a good place to share your rewarding experiences with others. Support groups for caregivers of people with Alzheimer's disease can take place in person or on an online message board.

Many organizations offer support groups for caregivers, including local hospitals and Alzheimer's groups like the Alzheimer's Association.

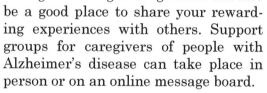

Caregivers can search for in-person support groups in their local communities or join an online support forum at the Alzheimer's Association's caregiver support page:

http://www.alz.org/apps/we_can_help/support_groups.asp.

The Alzheimer's Association offers online classes, as well as CDs and DVDs that give helpful information and help build caregiving skills. These resources are available at

http://www.alz.org/care/alzheimers-dementia-care-training-certification.asp

Disease-Related Education

Organizations like the Alzheimer's Association offer information, programs, and workshops on skills for caregiving and managing difficult behaviors. Caregiver training can help caregivers learn to handle the physical and mental challenges of caregiving better and to learn new skills. These skills can help improve stress levels and depression symptoms in caregivers.

Adult Day Care and Respite Services

Adult day care programs provide a safe place where people with Alzheimer's disease can stay during the day when their caregivers can't be available. Staff members take care of and provide activities for their clients, usually for an hourly fee.

To find an adult day care service near you, use the National Adult Day Services Association's locator at http://nadsa.org/locator/.

For care lasting from a few days to a few weeks, respite services are available in nursing homes or other places for people with Alzheimer's disease. This can enable you to take a break or go on vacation.

To find respite services near you, use the National Respite Locator Service at http://archrespite.org/respitelocator.

Meal Services

Some local groups provide hot meals to people with Alzheimer's disease for free or for a small fee. The person with Alzheimer's must qualify for the service based on local guidelines.

Visit the Eldercare Locator at www.eldercare.gov to find a meal service near you.

Home Health Care

Home health care agencies can send an aide or nurse to your home to help you care for a person with Alzheimer's disease. These people are usually paid by the hour and can stay for a few hours or around the clock. Ask your doctor for a recommendation, and be sure to check references.

When you are signing a home health care agreement, find out:

- if the service is licensed and accredited
- how much the services costs
- what is and isn't included
- how the aides' experience and backgrounds are checked
- whom you should contact if there is a problem

The National Institutes of Health also offers an online list of helpful resources, such as handbooks, memoirs, and documentaries about dealing with the stress of being a caregiver. The list can be accessed at http://www.nia.nih.gov/alzheimers/coping-emotions-and-stress-alzheimers-caregiving-resource-list

71. How can I communicate better with a person with Alzheimer's disease?

As Alzheimer's disease progresses, the ability to communicate declines. However, there are ways to enhance interaction with a person with Alzheimer's disease, such as by using body language, tone of voice, and facial expression to help him or her process verbal information. See Table 8.1 for more tips.

Table 8.1 Tips to Enhance Communication

Approach the person from the front and address him or her by name.
Speak slowly and clearly.
Talk *to* the person; avoid talking *about* the person, as if he or she weren't there.
Maintain eye contact. If the person is sitting or lying down, sit down to be at the same level.
Give visual cues. If you want the person to see or use a certain object, signify this by touching or pointing to it.
Use clear words and short sentences. Say the name of the object or action instead of saying "it" or "that."
Minimize distractions and noise. Turn off the TV or radio while you are talking.
Ask one question at a time and allow enough time for a response. If the person does not respond the first time, ask again.
Try to keep your tone of voice and your body language positive, open, and reassuring. Sometimes feelings of frustration or stress can be perceived as anger or hostility.
Keep talking even if the person can no longer speak. It will show you care.

SOURCE: "Communication and Alzheimer's," Alzheimer's Association, July 31, 2014, http://www.alz.org/care/dementia-communication-tips.asp.

SOURCE: "Education and Care," Alzheimer's Foundation of America, accessed July 31, 2014, http://www.alzfdn.org/EducationandCare/techniques.html.

72. How can I show someone with advanced Alzheimer's disease that I care?

Research suggests that even people with advanced Alzheimer's disease can find comfort from a loved one. Acts like holding hands, hugging, and giving a kiss can be meaningful in the moment, even if they are soon forgotten.

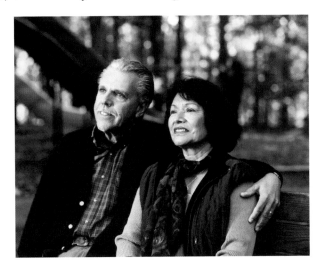

Other ways to show people with Alzheimer's disease you care include these:

- Playing their favorite music
- Reading books that are meaningful to them
- Looking at old photos together
- Brushing their hair
- Sitting outside together

73. How can I make the most of doctor's visits?

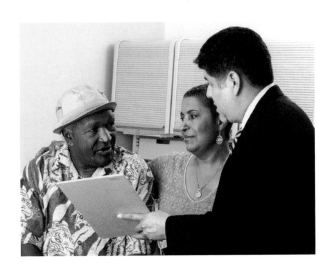

Caregivers play an essential role in helping to make sure that a person's needs are met, especially as symptoms progress. It's important to keep track of any changes in mood and abilities as they arise, so that they can be addressed at the next doctor's visit. An easy way to keep track of these events is through a care log.

To keep a care log, simply make a table that lists the date and time of an incident and then describe what happened. For example, "[Name of person with Alzheimer's] had a hard time sleeping tonight. [He or she] paced across the room for 2 hours. When I tried to get him to come to sleep he started to cry." Be sure to record any time a person with Alzheimer's shows depressive symptoms, behaves aggressively, or has a wandering incident. A care log is an easy way to let a doctor review the status of a person with Alzheimer's disease and meet his or her needs more effectively.

A medication log is also a useful tool to bring to each doctor's visit. It should list all current medications that the person is taking, including ones for Alzheimer's symptoms as well as other physical or psychological conditions; the side effects he or she has experienced; when the drugs were prescribed; and the instructions for their proper use.

Lastly, an appointment log can help you remember what issues or questions to bring up at the next doctor's appointment. On your appointment log, list the time and date of the next visit and write down the topics you want to address. Then take the appointment log with you and add recommendations (or to dos) to help address these concerns.

You can download templates for care, medication, and appointment logs from the Alzheimer's Association at

http://www.alz.org/alzheimers_disease_doctors_visit_checklist.asp

ON THE WEB

Here are some other helpful tips:

- Bring a snack, something to drink, and perhaps an activity to keep the person with Alzheimer's disease occupied while you wait for the appointment.
- Consider asking a friend or family member to accompany you to the appointment. This way, if you want to speak to the doctor in private for a moment, that person can assist you with caring for the patient.

1   "Caring for Someone," Alzheimers.gov, accessed July 31, 2014, http:// www.alzheimers.gov/caring.html.

2   Niklas Bergvall et al., "Relative importance of patient disease indicators and caregiver burden in Alzheimer's disease," *International Psychogeriatrics* 23, no. 1 (2011): 73–85.

3   James E. Galvin and Carl H. Sadowsky, "Practical Guidelines for the Recognition and Diagnosis of Dementia," *The Journal of the American Board of Family Medicine* 25, no. 3 (2012): 367–82. http://www.jabfm .org/content/25/3/367.long.

4   "Occupational Therapy Practice Guidelines for Adults with Alzheimer's Disease and Related Disorders," National Guideline Clearinghouse, accessed June 2, 2014, http://www.guideline.gov/content.aspx?id=16321 &search=alzheimer%27s+disease.

5   Helen C. Kales, Laura N. Gitlin, Constantine G. Lyketsos, and the Detroit Expert Panel on the Assessment and Management of the Neuropsychiatric Symptoms of Dementia, "Management of Neuropsychiatric Symptoms of Dementia in Clinical Settings: Recommendations from a Multidisciplinary Expert Panel," *Journal of the American Geriatrics Society* 62, no. 4 (2014): 762–9. http:// onlinelibrary.wiley.com/doi/10.1111/jgs.12730/abstract.

6   Constantine G. Lyketsos et al., "Neuropsychiatric Symptoms in Alzheimer's Disease," *Alzheimer's & Dementia: The Journal of the Alzheimer's Association* 7, no. 5 (2011): 532–9. www. alzheimersanddementia.com/article/S1552-5260(11)02575-1/abstract.

7   Somaia Mohamed et al., "Caregiver burden in Alzheimer's disease: Cross-sectional and longitudinal patient correlates," *American Journal of Geriatric Psychiatry* 18, no. 10 (2010): 917-27.

8   "Caring for Someone with Alzheimers--Taking Care of Yourself," NIHSeniorHealth, last updated December 2012, accessed July 31, 2014, http://nihseniorhealth.gov/alzheimerscare/selfcare/01.html.

9   "Middle-Stage Caregiving," Alzheimer's Association, accessed July 31, 2014, http://www.alz.org/care/alzheimers-mid-moderate-stage-caregiving.asp.

10 "Communication Tips & Techniques," Alzheimer's Association, accessed July 31, 2014, http://www.alz.org/texascapital/in_my_ community_14326.asp.

11 "Caring for Someone with Alzheimers--Help with Home Care," NIHSeniorHealth, last updated December 2012, accessed July 31, 2014, http://nihseniorhealth.gov/alzheimerscare/helpwithhomecare/ 01.html.

12   "Caregiver Guide: Tips for Caregivers of People with Alzheimer's Disease," National Institute on Aging, last updated June 4, 2014, accessed July 31, 2014, http://www.nia.nih.gov/alzheimers/publication/caregiver-guide.

13   "Communication and Alzheimer's," Alzheimer's Association, accessed July 31, 2014, http://www.alz.org/care/dementia-communication-tips.asp.

14   "Education and Care," Alzheimer's Foundation of America, accessed July 31, 2014, http://www.alzfdn.org/EducationandCare/techniques.html.

15   "Late-Stage Caregiving," Alzheimer's Association, accessed July 31, 2014, http://www.alz.org/care/alzheimers-late-end-stage-caregiving.asp.

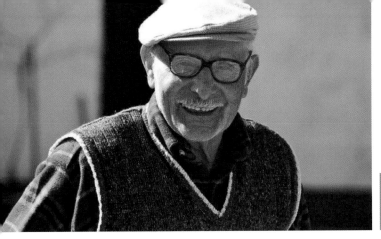

Planning Ahead

Case Study

When Violet needed more care than her daughters and husband could provide, they moved her to a licensed elder care facility. Located just a few blocks from her long-time home, the residential facility provides 24-hour care for up to five people at a time. Her daughters and husband visit her as often as they can, especially in the mornings, when she is most alert and most likely to recognize them. The facility provides Violet everything she needs, including hygiene, grooming, and mobility assistance. One of the benefits that her family didn't expect was that staff at the facility helped them talk through and make decisions about the next steps in Violet's care, including end-of-life planning and "do not resuscitate" orders.

74. Why plan ahead?

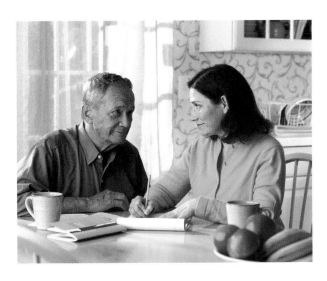

Living with a progressive disease involves the need for financial resources and access to health care. It may also bring up some legal issues that need to be addressed. People with Alzheimer's disease should be involved in planning for their future, including finding the right kinds of services and deciding on ways to pay for them. If these needs are planned for early enough, people with Alzheimer's disease can play a part in the decisions that will affect their lives down the road.

On the other hand, not planning ahead may limit the options for care, services, and support that are available when the need for them arises. If the planning process is delayed, then the person with Alzheimer's disease may not have the ability to have a voice in the decisions that are made for his or her own care.

The Alzheimer's Association offers the Alzheimer's Navigator, an online tool to help you create a personalized action plan for managing Alzheimer's disease and to link you with information, support, and local resources. Visit

https://www.alzheimersnavigator.org.

ON THE WEB

Delaying the process of planning may also place undue stress on the friends and family members of a person with Alzheimer's disease. Providing care and support to a loved one with Alzheimer's disease can be stressful already, and facing the issues involved in planning can feel like adding more stress, but taking the time to make a long-term plan as soon as possible can help reduce this anxiety.

75. What legal and financial matters should I consider?

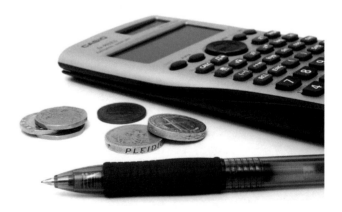

At some point, a person with Alzheimer's disease will no longer be able to manage his or her financial affairs. **Advance directives** for financial and estate management are documents that ensure that late-stage or end-of-life financial decisions are carried out as he or she wishes.

An advance directive for financial and estate management may include a will, a durable power of attorney for finances, and a living trust. They should be created when the person with Alzheimer's disease is still able to make decisions.

Will

A will states how a person's money, possessions, and property will be shared when the person dies. A will is similar to a living trust but typically covers only how a person's estate will be split up after his or her death. In a will, a person can designate an executor, or someone who will see that the estate is distributed in accordance with the will. A will can also designate relatives or non-family members such as godchildren or stepchildren to inherit some of a person's estate. In the absence of a will or a trust, the state's court system will determine which family members are beneficiaries of a person's assets. This usually includes only spouses, biological children, and siblings.

Durable Power of Attorney

A durable power of attorney gives someone who is selected the power to make decisions about financial matters when the person with Alzheimer's disease is no longer capable to make these decisions. A durable power of attorney is enacted by filling out and signing a form, which is specific to each state. One person can be chosen to have power of attorney for all financial matters, or different people can be selected for different responsibilities, such as selling a house. Durable powers of attorney may give a person different rights depending on the state in which the document is signed.

Living Trust

A living trust is a document that gives instructions about the person's estate and appoints a trustee to hold and distribute property and funds on the person's behalf. It determines how a person's estate will be used both before and after his or her death. A living trust states how a person wants his or her assets to be used, even when that person can no longer communicate these wishes. For instance, a living trust can state how assets will be used to pay for health care and nursing home fees, as well as who will be the beneficiaries of the estate when the person passes away. Generally, the larger a person's estate, the more he or she needs a living trust.

Having a living trust may help avoid the probate process, which is the court's way of splitting up a person's estate after his or her death.

A lawyer is not necessary to create a living trust, a will, or to designate a person to have durable power of attorney. For people with just a few assets to manage, a simple trust or will can be written and notarized without hiring a lawyer. However, the more assets a person has, the more useful it is to hire a lawyer to oversee the estate planning process. A lawyer can give valuable insight into state and federal tax laws and help you get the most out of your plan.

Elder law attorneys specialize in helping families understand their financial options and plan to see that their wishes are carried out.

76. What financial records should be shared with caregivers?

It's a good idea to put financial records in order early in the disease process. Share the following information with the person who will be managing your finances:

- Income sources and assets, including any pensions, IRAs, 401(k)s, and interest from these and other accounts
- Social security and Medicare information
- Insurance policy names and numbers, including car, disability, health, home, life, and long-term care insurance
- Bank account names and numbers, including checking, savings, and credit union accounts
- Investment income and stockbrokers' names and phone numbers
- Copy of your most recent tax return
- Location of your most recent will
- Records of any liabilities, including property tax
- Information on how and when mortgages and debts are paid
- Location of original deed of trust for your home and of car title and registration
- Credit and debit card names and numbers
- Location of safe deposit box and key

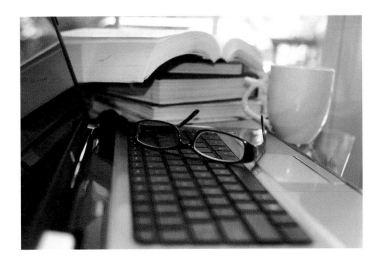

Advance directives for health care are documents that enable people with Alzheimer's disease to ensure that their health care wishes will be followed, even when they are no longer to able to communicate or make decisions. An advance directive can be amended or added to as long as the person still has the capacity to make decisions about his or her future care. Typically, it includes the following documents.

Living Will

A living will states how you would like to be treated in a life-threatening emergency, including the procedures you would want, the ones you would not want, and the situations under which each applies. These procedures include the use of cardiopulmonary resuscitation (CPR), ventilators, feeding tubes and intravenous (IV) fluids, and comfort care. For example, a living will would state if you want a feeding tube to give you nutrition when you can no longer feed yourself.

Durable Power of Attorney for Health Care

This is a legal document that names someone who will make medical decisions for you when you are no longer able to. This person is called a "health care proxy," "surrogate," or "agent." A durable power of attorney can be made in addition to or in place of a living will.

A health care proxy should be someone you trust to make sure that your wishes and needs are met during the later stages of the disease. Your health care proxy needs to understand your treatment goals, values, and beliefs well enough to communicate them to doctors, caretakers, and loved ones. It also helps to select someone who can stay calm during a crisis and who can be assertive when standing up for your medical needs and wishes.

It is a good idea to name a back-up health care proxy in case the primary proxy cannot be present when needed. If a health care proxy has not been designated by a person with Alzheimer's disease, the state's laws will dictate who will make medical care decisions on his or her behalf. Depending on the state, this may be a family member or it may be a doctor or hospital worker.

The American Bar Association has compiled a list of helpful resources that can guide people with Alzheimer's disease and their loved ones through the process of creating advance care directives. It can be accessed here:

ON THE WEB

http://www.americanbar.org/content/dam/aba/administrative/law_aging/Health_Decisions_Resources.pdf.

Other Advance Care Planning Documents

You can also prepare separate documents regarding "do not resuscitate" orders, organ and tissue donation, dialysis, and blood transfusion, which may not be covered in a living will.

78. What long-term residential care options exist?

"Long-term care" refers to a range of services and supports that help a person who has Alzheimer's disease with activities of daily living, such as getting dressed, eating, bathing, and doing housework. Most long-term care is not medical care but personal care. Long-term care services can be provided at home or in a long-term care facility. When a person with Alzheimer's disease can no longer be cared for safely at home, relatives often consider moving him or her to facility-based, or residential, care.

Assisted Living

People in the earlier stages of Alzheimer's disease may want to continue to live independently for as long as possible but also to have access to services that make activities of daily living easier. In this case, assisted living may be a good option to consider. In assisted living facilities, people with Alzheimer's disease, seniors, and other people with difficulties taking care of themselves can live independently in a housing community that offers assistance with housekeeping, meals, taking medicine, and activities. Residents usually pay monthly rent plus the cost of any medical and nursing services.

Continuing Care Retirement Communities

Continuing care retirement communities feature a range of housing options that enable residents to access increasing levels of care as they need it. Usually located on a single campus, a continuing care retirement community has independent community living, assisted living, and nursing home care. For people in the earlier stages of Alzheimer's disease, living in one of these communities can help ease the transition from independent to assisted living.

Nursing Homes

Nursing homes provide the same services that are found in an assisted living facility but also provide full-time nursing care around the clock. Nursing homes are also called skilled nursing facilities, long-term care facilities, and custodial care facilities.

By age 80, 75 percent of people with Alzheimer's disease will reside in a nursing home, compared with only 4 percent of the general population.

Some nursing homes have special care units that are designed to meet the needs of patients with a specific condition. The ones for people with Alzheimer's disease and other types of dementia are sometimes called "memory care units" and may include specially trained staff and enhanced security to prevent wandering.

To learn more about long-term care, visit

http://longtermcare.gov.

79. What is end-of-life care?

"End-of-life care" refers to the support and medical care that is given during the time surrounding death. Ideally, during the early stages of Alzheimer's disease there should be a talk about values, preferences, and goals related to death and dying, because in many cases people can be living and dying for days, weeks, or months. While some people may wish to be kept alive and comfortable as long as medically possible, others may prefer to live only with a certain level of quality of life, even if it means a shorter life.

Hospice care is usually provided for people who are expected to live six or fewer months. The goal of hospice care is to provide peace, comfort, and dignity. Hospice caregivers work to control pain and other symptoms to help the person be as comfortable as possible. They also provide services to support the person's family members. Hospice care can take place at home or in a hospice center, hospital, or skilled nursing facility.

Palliative care provides treatment for the discomfort, symptoms, and stress of Alzheimer's disease. It can be provided at any point during an illness but is always provided as part of hospice care.

When discussing end-of-life care, talk about and make clear to your loved ones and caregivers:

- Where you want to spend your last days
- What a "good death" means to you
- Whether you would want tube feeding and ventilation
- Whether you would want to be resuscitated (receive CPR) if your heart stopped
- Whether you want any medicines or life-prolonging treatments to be stopped at a certain point

Then create health care advance directives to make sure that your wishes are followed. (For more information about health care advance directives, see Question 77 What are health care advance directives?).

 References

1 "Revocable Trusts | Section of Real Property, Trust and Estate Law," American Bar Association, accessed August 1, 2014, http://www .americanbar.org/groups/real_property_trust_estate/resources/estate_ planning/revocable_trusts.html.

2 "Legal Steps for Financial Well-Being--Long-Term Care Information," LongTermCare.gov accessed, August 1, 2014 http://longtermcare.gov/ how-to-decide/legal-steps-for-financial-well-being/.

3 "An Introduction to Wills | Section of Real Property, Trust and Estate Law," American Bar Association, accessed August 1, 2014, http://www .americanbar.org/groups/real_property_trust_estate/resources/estate_ planning/an_introduction_to_wills.html.

4 "Legal and Financial Planning for People with Alzheimer's Disease Fact Sheet," National Institute on Aging, last updated May 2, 2014, accessed May 29, 2014, http://www.nia.nih.gov/alzheimers/publication/legal-and-financial-planning-people-alzheimers-disease-fact-sheet.

5 "Getting Your Affairs in Order," National Institute on Aging, last updated May 6, 2014, accessed July 31, 2014, http://www.nia.nih.gov/health/publication/getting-your-affairs-order.

6 "Advance Care Planning," National Institute on Aging, last updated July 18, 2014, accessed July 31, 2014, http://www.nia.nih.gov/health/publication/advance-care-planning.

7 "Health Care Proxies," Medicare Interactive, accessed August 1, 2014, http://www.medicareinteractive.org/page2.php?topic=counselor&page=script&script_id=1335.

8 "Assisted Living Options | Assisted Living Homes & Elder Care Options | Long Term Care Options in Assisted Living," Assisted Living Federation of America, accessed August 1, 2014, http://www.alfa.org/alfa/Senior_Living_Options.asp.

9 "Assisted Living - Long-Term Care Information," LongTermCare. gov, accessed August 1, 2014 http://longtermcare.gov/where-you-live-matters/living-in-a-facility/assisted-living/.

10 "Continuing Care Retirement Communities--Long-Term Care Information," LongTermCare.gov, accessed August 1, 2014, http://longtermcare.gov/where-you-live-matters/living-in-a-facility/continuing-care-retirement-communities/

11 "Residential Care | Caregiver Center," Alzheimer's Association, accessed August 1, 2014, http://www.alz.org/care/alzheimers-dementia-residential-facilities.asp.

12 "2014 Alzheimer's Disease Facts and Figures," Alzheimer's Association, accessed March 31, 2014, http://www.alz.org/downloads/facts_figures_2014.pdf.

13 "Hospice Care," MedlinePlus, last updated July 17, 2014, accessed August 1, 2014, http://www.nlm.nih.gov/medlineplus/hospicecare.html.

14 "Palliative Care," MedlinePlus, last updated July 7, 2014, accessed August 1, 2014, http://www.nlm.nih.gov/medlineplus/palliativecare.html.

Appendix: Resources

There are many organizations that help people with Alzheimer's disease, their loved ones, and caregivers. Contact them for information, assistance, and support.

Alzheimer's Association

National voluntary health organization committed to finding a cure for Alzheimer's disease and helping those affected by it. The Alzheimer's Association is a nonprofit organization offering information and support services to people with Alzheimer's disease and their families.

Alzheimer's Association
225 North Michigan Avenue
Floor 17
Chicago, IL 60601-7633
info@alz.org
http://www.alz.org
Telephone: 800-272-3900 (24-hour helpline), TDD: 312-335-5886
Fax: 866-699-1246

Alzheimer's Disease Education and Referral Center (ADEAR)

The National Institute on Aging's ADEAR Center offers information and publications in English and Spanish for families, caregivers, and professionals on diagnosis, treatment, patient care, caregiver needs, long-term care, education and training, and research related to Alzheimer's disease. Staff can refer you to local and national resources. The Center is a service of the National Institute on Aging, part of the federal government's National Institutes of Health.

Alzheimer's Disease Education and Referral Center (ADEAR)
National Institute on Aging
P.O. Box 8250
Silver Spring, MD 20907-8250
adear@nia.nih.gov
http://www.nia.nih.gov/alzheimers
Telephone: 800-438-4380
Fax: 301-495-3334

Alzheimer's Foundation of America

This foundation works to provide optimal care and services to individuals confronting dementia and to their caregivers and families through member organizations dedicated to improving quality of life. Services include a toll-free hotline, publications and other materials, conferences, and workshops.

Alzheimer's Foundation of America
322 Eighth Avenue
7th Floor
New York, NY 10001
info@alzfdn.org
http://www.alzfdn.org
Telephone: 866-232-8484)
Fax: 646-638-1546

BrightFocus Foundation

A nonprofit charitable organization dedicated to funding research and educating the public on Alzheimer's disease, glaucoma, and macular degeneration.

BrightFocus Foundation
22512 Gateway Center Drive
Clarksburg, MD 20871
info@brightfocus.org
http://www.brightfocus.org/alzheimers/
Telephone: 800-437-2423
Fax: 301-258-9454

Children of Aging Parents

This nonprofit group provides information, referrals, publications, and conferences for adult children caring for their older parents. Caregivers of people with Alzheimer's disease also may find these resources helpful.

Children of Aging Parents
P.O. Box 167
Richboro, PA 18954
Telephone: 800-227-7294
www.caps4caregivers.org

Eldercare Locator

This public service of the U.S. Administration on Aging connects families to community resources, such as home care, adult day care, and nursing homes.

Eldercare Locator
Telephone: 800-677-1116
eldercarelocator@n4a.org
http://www.eldercare.gov.

Family Caregiver Alliance/ National Center on Caregiving

Supports and assists families and caregivers of adults with debilitating health conditions. Offers programs and consultation on caregiving issues at local, state, and national levels. Offers free publications and support online, including a national directory of publicly funded caregiver support programs.

Family Caregiver Alliance/National Center on Caregiving
785 Market St.
Suite 750
San Francisco, CA 94103
info@caregiver.org
http://www.caregiver.org
Telephone: 415-434-3388, 800-445-8106
Fax: 415-434-3508

National Family Caregivers Association

Grassroots organization dedicated to supporting and improving the lives of America's family caregivers. Created to educate, support, empower, and advocate for the millions of Americans who care for their ill, aged, or disabled loved ones.

National Family Caregivers Association
10400 Connecticut Avenue
Suite 500
Kensington, MD 20895-3944
info@thefamilycaregiver.org
http://www.thefamilycaregiver.org
Telephone: 800-896-3650
Fax: 301-942-2302

National Hospice and Palliative Care Organization

Nonprofit membership organization representing hospice and palliative care programs and professionals. Provides free referrals to the public for hospice listings across the United States and internationally. Distributes free packets of general information describing hospice services and the Medicare Hospice Benefit.

National Hospice and Palliative Care Organization
1731 King Street
Alexandria, VA 22314
nhpco_info@nhpco.org
http://www.nhpco.org
Telephone: 703-837-1500, 800-658-8898 (helpline)
Fax: 703-837-1233

Well Spouse Association

International nonprofit, volunteer-based organization whose mission is to provide emotional support to, raise consciousness about, and advocate for the spouses/partners of the chronically ill and/or disabled.

Well Spouse Association
63 West Main Street
Suite H
Freehold, NJ 07728
info@wellspouse.org
http://www.wellspouse.org
Telephone: 800-838-0879, 732-577-8899
Fax: 732-577-8644

Index